Wound Care Nursing

A Guide to Practice

Other titles by Ausmed Publications

Gastrostomy Care: A Guide to Practice
Edited by Catherine Barrett
Available as audiobook and textbook

Nursing Documentation in Aged Care: A Guide to Practice
Edited by Christine Crofton and Gaye Witney
Available as audiobook and textbook

Nurse Managers: A Guide to Practice
Edited by Andrew Crowther
Available as audiobook and textbook

Aged Care Nursing: A Guide to Practice
Edited by Susan Carmody and Sue Forster
Available as audiobook and textbook

Dementia Nursing: A Guide to Practice
Edited by Rosalie Hudson
Available as audiobook and textbook

Palliative Care Nursing: A Guide to Practice (2nd edn)
Edited by Margaret O'Connor and Sanchia Aranda

Lymphoedema
Edited by Robert Twycross, Karen Jenns, and Jacquelyne Todd

Communicating with Dying People and their Relatives
Jean Lugton

How Drugs Work
Hugh McGavock

Evidence-based Management
Rosemary Stewart

Communication and the Manager's Job
Annie Phillips

Assertiveness and the Manager's Job
Annie Phillips

Renal Nursing—A Practical Approach
Bobbee Terrill

Ageing at Home--Practical Approaches to Community Care
Edited by Theresa Cluning

Complementary Therapies in Nursing and Midwifery
Edited by Pauline McCabe

Keeping in Touch--with someone who has Alzheimer's
Jane Crisp

Geriatric Medicine--a pocket guide for doctors, nurses, other health professionals and students (2nd edn)
Len Gray, Michael Woodward, Ron Scholes, David Fonda & Wendy Busby

Living Dying Caring--life and death in a nursing home
Rosalie Hudson & Jennifer Richmond

Caring for People with Problem Behaviours (2nd edn)
Bernadette Keane & Carolyn Dixon

Practical Approaches to Infection Control in Residential Aged Care (2nd edn)
Kevin Kendall

Spirituality—the heart of nursing
Edited by Susan Ronaldson

All of these titles are available from the publisher:
Ausmed Publications
277 Mt Alexander Road, Ascot Vale, Melbourne, Victoria 3032, Australia
website: <www.ausmed.com.au>
email: <ausmed@ausmed.com.au>

Wound Care Nursing
A Guide to Practice

Edited by Sue Templeton

Foreword by Jan Rice

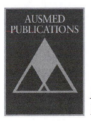

AUSMED PUBLICATIONS
MELBOURNE – SEATTLE

Copyright ©Ausmed Publications Pty Ltd 2005

Ausmed Publications Pty Ltd
Melbourne – Seattle

Melbourne office:
277 Mt Alexander Road
Ascot Vale, Melbourne, Victoria 3032, Australia
ABN 49 824 739 129
Telephone: + 61 3 9375 7311
Fax: + 61 3 9375 7299
email: <ausmed@ausmed.com.au>
website: <www.ausmed.com.au>

Seattle office:
Martin P. Hill Consulting
157 Yesler Way, Suite 300
Seattle, Washington 98104
USA
Tel: 206-624-6609
Fax: 206-624-6707
Mobile: 415-309-2338
email: <mphill@mphconsult.com>

Although the Publisher has taken every care to ensure the accuracy of the professional, clinical, and technical components of this publication, it accepts no responsibility for any loss or damage suffered by any person as a result of following the procedures described or acting on information set out in this publication. The Publisher reminds readers that the information in this publication is no substitute for individual medical and/or nursing assessment and treatment by professional staff.

Wound Care Nursing: A Guide to Practice
ISBN 0 9750445 1 6
First published by Ausmed Publications Pty Ltd, 2005.
Reprinted 2005

National Library of Australia Cataloguing-in-Publication data
        Wound care nursing : a guide to practice.

        Bibliography.
        Includes index.
        ISBN 0 9750445 1 6.

        1. Wounds and injuries - Nursing. 2. Wound healing. I.
        Templeton, Sue.

        617.1

Produced by Ginross Publishing
Printed in China

Contents

Dedication

This book is dedicated to all nurses who bring their knowledge, skills, and professionalism to the care of wounded people.

Foreword

Jan Rice

It is with pleasure that I write this foreword for *Wound Care Nursing: A Guide To Practice*. There is no doubt that wound care extends across all sectors of nursing. There is also no question that things have changed in wound-care nursing—for the better.

It is important that knowledge of wound-care nursing is readily available to nurses. Many healthcare authorities are experiencing nursing shortages, and nurses are often required to teach others about wound care. This book will meet this need. The book avoids complexity, without being simplistic. It is comprehensive, without being too lengthy. Above all, it is practical.

Each of the chapter authors provides a concise understanding of the approaches needed in particular specialties, while always being aware of the wounded patient as a person. The editor of the book, Sue Templeton, sets the scene in Chapter 1, which emphasises the feelings of a wounded person and the importance of recognising the person beyond the wound. Whether dealing with a trauma wound, or a malignant lesion, or a lower-leg ulcer, the approach taken by the chapter authors is consistent—starting with the patient's perception of the impact of the wound on his or her life, then ascertaining the precise aetiology of the wound, and then following an accepted clinical pathway in managing the wounded person.

Wound-care nursing is now beginning to receive the recognition it deserves. The book highlights wound management as a developing speciality in its own right, but still manages to extend basic knowledge without being too prescriptive or specialised. Rather, the book highlights the *principles* of practice—and encourages readers to think about their current practice. While being aware of more sophisticated knowledge and practices, the book promotes the notion that simplicity is a virtue.

This book should be recommended reading for all general nurses. The style of writing encourages the reader to explore and think. The layout of the text is uncluttered, and easy to read.

As an educator in this field, I can only say that my job will be made easier if all those engaging in wound care read this book and absorb the excellent information it provides.

Jan Rice

Jan Rice is a registered nurse, registered midwife, and wound nurse consultant who holds a certificate in plastic and reconstructive-surgery nursing. She is on several editorial advisory boards and frequently writes for wound journals. Jan has been the driving force behind Wound Foundation of Australia (Monash University). This foundation spreads knowledge about the principles and practice of wound care to healthcare professionals and carers throughout Australia and internationally, specifically in the South Pacific. This education ensures that best-practice principles are put in place and that patients are well informed about the newer technologies. Jan is also manager of the wound clinic at Austin Health. This clinic has been operating for 10 years and provides wound-care advice for people from all over Victoria (Australia).

Preface

Sue Templeton

Nurses and wound management

The management of persons with wounds is an interesting, challenging, and rewarding endeavour. Wound management is practised by nurses in all care settings with patients of all ages. At some time, nurses who work in settings as diverse as a residential aged-care facility, an intensive-care unit of a major hospital, or a small clinic in a remote rural community can all expect to manage a person with a wound.

Wounds are thus a common and significant cause of morbidity and mortality—and represent a financial and social burden to individuals and the wider community.

'At some time, all nurses can expect to manage a person with a wound.'

Nurses have a vital role in wound management. Because they spend so much time with patients, nurses are well positioned to assess and implement wound-management interventions to achieve optimal outcomes. Through a close professional relationship with patients, nurses can deliver evidence-based wound management with a person-centred focus. The apparently simple act of changing a dressing epitomises the caring nature of nursing—the healing touch of a nurse in reaching out to a wounded person.

Wound management is both a generalist and a specialist skill. Because virtually all nurses care for a person with a wound at some stage during their careers, wound management is a generalist skill. Every nurse must be able to plan and implement interventions that facilitate optimal outcomes and cause no harm. Basic skills in wound management are thus an essential aspect of sound general nursing. In addition to these generalist skills, some nurses have developed advanced skills in wound management.

'Nurses have built a significant reputation as expert wound-management clinicians in their own right.'

These nurses might hold a position as a wound-management specialist, consultant, or resource nurse. The development of advanced nursing roles provides nurses with an opportunity to build a career in wound management.

The scientific and technological advances that are now being made in wound management have the potential to revolutionise the treatment of wounds. As a consequence, wound management as a specialty area of practice has burgeoned in recent years. There are now many local, national, and international associations that are dedicated to the pursuit of excellence in wound management. Multidisciplinary associations for wound management meet regularly to debate contemporary issues and to develop wound-management guidelines and documents. This collaboration of expert clinicians, researchers, and scientists provides a powerful unifying voice for wound management. In parallel with these developments, the role of nurses has also seen significant development. Nurses are no longer valued only for their skills in bandage application; rather, nurses have built a significant reputation as expert wound-management clinicians in their own right.

The need for a nursing text

Despite the proliferation of knowledge in modern wound management, there are still many settings in which wound-management education and resources are not readily available. And because wound management is an ancient and widely practised craft, many practices have developed that are based on tradition, outdated techniques, and obsolete knowledge.

Contemporary journals and guidelines might not be available to nurses in their workplaces, and, in some areas, opportunities to attend educational sessions are limited.

For these reasons, and others, many nurses lack confidence when caring for persons with wounds. It is sometimes difficult for nurses to know whether the treatment being carried out is supported by evidence and accepted as best practice. To optimise outcomes for persons with wounds, nurses require an understanding of basic anatomy and physiology, the processes involved in normal healing, and the factors that can delay wound healing. In addition, they require skill in dressings and other interventions that promote wound healing.

'This book is written by nurses for nurses in a clear style that facilitates the application of practical knowledge in the clinical setting.'

Wound Care Nursing: A Guide to Practice sets out to meet these daunting needs. The book is written predominantly by nurses for nurses in a clear style that facilitates the application of practical knowledge in the clinical setting.

The aims of *Wound Care Nursing: A Guide to Practice* are:

- to explain the basic physiology of wounding and healing;
- to discuss the pathophysiology and management of the most common types of wounds;
- to provide contemporary information based on evidence and clinical experience;
- to provide practical, relevant information that can be readily applied to practice; and
- to discuss contemporary developments and concepts in wound management.

The authors of the chapters are nurses and other health professionals who are acknowledged experts in various fields. All are dedicated to working with patients to ensure that they achieve the best outcomes with the least impact on their quality of life. All have welcomed this opportunity to enhance the understanding and proficiency of nurses in wound management.

Celebrating achievement

Wound Care Nursing: A Guide to Practice has been written to 'de-mystify' wound management, and to encourage nurses to strive for excellence in their practice. This book will benefit all nurses in all practice settings—including those working in acute care, residential aged care, and community care. Nurses in metropolitan, rural, and remote practice settings will all find this book invaluable.

> *'Through this book, nurses are encouraged to celebrate and take pride in their achievements as caring professionals who make a profound and positive difference to people's lives.'*

Through *Wound Care Nursing: A Guide to Practice*, nurses will increase their theoretical knowledge and their practical skills. They will become empowered in caring for persons with a variety of wounds.

The authors trust that colleagues who read this book will achieve confidence and success in their wound management. Through this book, nurses are encouraged to celebrate and take pride in their achievements as caring professionals who make a profound and positive difference to people's lives.

About the Authors

Keryln Carville
Chapter 16

Keryln Carville is a registered nurse who holds postgraduate qualifications in stomal-therapy nursing. Her PhD thesis was entitled: 'The Evolution and Experience of Stomal Therapy Nurses in Australia'. Keryln is nurse clinical consultant in wound and ostomy management for Silver Chain (Western Australia), and she holds an adjunct appointment as associate professor of domiciliary nursing at Curtin University (Western Australia) where she has developed and coordinates postgraduate studies in domiciliary nursing. She is a founding and life member of the Western Australia Wound Care Association. Keryln was awarded a Churchill Fellowship in 1995 to review clinical practice, education, and research in wound management in the United States and Britain. She is the current editor of the *Journal of Stomal Therapy Australia* and an editorial board member of *Primary Intention* and the *ACCNS Journal for Community Nurses*. Keryln has a broad clinical practice and lectures in wound and ostomy management at an undergraduate and postgraduate level, both nationally and internationally. She has a particular interest in chronic wound management and has an increasing commitment to research in the field.

Therese Chand
Chapter 5

After finishing a bachelor's degree in nursing from the University of the Philippines, Therese Chand worked in the emergency room of the University of the Philippines/ Philippines General Hospital. She migrated to Australia in 1997. Therese has worked as a paediatric nurse at the Royal Alexandra Hospital for Children (Sydney, Australia) and as a clinical nurse consultant specialising in stomal therapy, tracheostomy care, and wound management. She has a special interest in nursing education and has lectured at the NSW College of Nursing, at the University of Sydney, and in the community. Therese has facilitated seminars and study days on wound management and stomal therapy. She has published several papers in nursing journals and was recipient of the Nurses Publication Award in 2003 (Children's Hospital Medical Council). Therese was a member of a nursing team that received an innovation award from the NSW Department of Health for a project that reduced the incidence of pressure areas in children. In addition to her nursing degree, Therese holds a graduate diploma in health science (nurse education), a certificate in stomal therapy, and a certificate in ICU/CCU nursing.

Tazmin Clingan
Chapter 14

Tazmin Clingan is a registered nurse and podiatrist who holds bachelor's degrees in nursing and applied science (podiatry). After working in private practice, Tazmin joined the Multidisciplinary High Risk Foot Clinic in the Diabetes Centre of the Royal Prince Alfred Hospital (Sydney, Australia). Her role includes the identification and management of high-risk foot problems in people with diabetes. Tazmin is also involved with the Diabetes Amputation Prevention Program through which she delivers education to nurses and general practitioners about foot disease in people with diabetes.

Taliesin Ellis
Chapter 19

Taliesin Ellis is a lecturer in the School of Nursing and Midwifery, University of South Australia. He has been involved in teaching and the practice of wound management for 18 years, specialising in dressing procedure and development of educational programs. Tal was a founding member of the South Australian Wound Management Association, and was its inaugural president. He was also a founding member of the Australian Wound Management Association, and was its inaugural secretary. He practises and consults in wound management in older people, and is a consultant to the wound-management industry at large. Tal co-developed the University of South Australia's online wound management course in 1998 and is still the coordinator of this course. He is the co-author of the 'Wound Field Concept'. His research interests include the evidence base for dressing procedures, skin tears, pressure ulcers, managing wounds in older people, and IT-based wound-management advances.

Sheila Kavanagh
Chapter 13

Sheila Kavanagh is a registered nurse and midwife who holds a degree in nursing and an operating room certificate. Sheila did her initial training at Whyalla Hospital (South

Australia) where she also completed her midwifery training and worked in operating theatres. Following a family move to Adelaide (South Australia), Sheila commenced work at the Royal Adelaide Hospital Burns Unit as the unit operating-room nurse. She has been the nurse in charge of the unit since 1996. Sheila is an active member of the Australian & New Zealand Burn Association (ANZBA), having served as state representative, treasurer, and vice-president. She is also a member of ANZBA education committee and is a key instructor for the ANZBA's national course in the emergency management of severe burns. Sheila was a member of the Royal Adelaide Hospital Burns Assessment team that was sent to Darwin to assist in the care of the survivors of the Bali bombing. In 2003, Sheila received a nursing excellence award in nursing clinical practice. She is one of the founders of the Julian Burton Burns Trust, which has been set up to raise money for the Royal Adelaide Burns Unit.

Linda Kilworth
Chapter 7

Linda Kilworth is a dietitian and nutritionist who has worked for more than twelve years as a consultant to various residential-care facilities in Brisbane and south-east Queensland (Australia). Her role is to advise on nutrition, dietary planning, food-service management, and food standards. Linda is involved in developing policies and procedures, communicating these to the relevant staff members, and developing processes of review and evaluation. This consultancy also encompasses call-outs to various residential aged-care facilities to conduct individual dietary assessments and advice, to develop nutrition-screening methods, and to provide practical advice on dietary modifications.

Avril Lunken
Chapter 17

Avril Lunken trained and worked in the United Kingdom as a community occupational therapist. In the past eight years in Australia she has worked in aged care, especially residential aged care. Avril has undertaken additional training in the Vodder method of manual lymph drainage (MLD) and in complex decongestive therapy—which qualifies her to treat a wide range of conditions, including lymphoedema. In her private practice, Avril has a special interest in early intervention for women who have been treated for breast cancer. Avril is an accredited member of the Australian Association of Occupational Therapists, MLD (UK), Lymphoedema Practitioners Education Group of Victoria, Australasian Lymphology Association, and the Lymphoedema Association of Australia.

Pam Morey
Chapters 8 and 9

Pam Morey has been a clinical nurse consultant in wound management at Sir Charles Gairdner Hospital (Perth, Western Australia) for the past eight years. Her background includes 12 years working in plastic and orthopaedic surgery—including emergency, elective, and reconstructive surgery. She holds a certificate in stomal therapy and a post-graduate diploma in clinical specialisation. She has recently registered to practise as a nurse practitioner and is completing a master's degree. Pam's areas of interest include all wound types—particularly complex and challenging wounds, skin tears, leg ulcers, and pressure-ulcer prevention and management. She has been involved extensively in wound-care education within the hospital setting as part of her professional affiliations. Pam is the vice-president of the Western Australian Wound Care Association and state representative to the Australian Wound Management Association. She won the Western Australian Nursing Board Nursing Excellence awards for Metropolitan Acute Care Nurse and Nurse of the Year in 2003.

Wayne Naylor
Chapter 15

Wayne Naylor is a New Zealand registered nurse who began his career in forensic psychiatry before moving into general surgery, and then to reconstructive plastic surgery and burns. After a move to the United Kingdom, Wayne worked at the Royal Marsden Hospital in London where he gained further qualifications in cancer nursing. For a little over three years Wayne was employed as the wound-management research nurse at the Marsden, a role that involved research, clinical patient care, education, and quality-assurance activities related to wound management in cancer patients. Wayne has published several journal articles and book chapters, and was lead editor for the *Royal Marsden Hospital Handbook of Wound Management in Cancer Care*. He also contributed a chapter on malignant wounds to the Ausmed publication *Palliative Care Nursing: A Guide to Practice*. Wayne now works as a clinical nurse specialist at the Wellington Cancer Centre in New Zealand. He has a special interest in the management of wounds related to cancer and cancer therapies, including malignant wounds, radiotherapy skin reactions, and cutaneous graft versus host disease.

Jenny Prentice
Chapter 12

Jenny Prentice completed her training as a registered general and obstetric nurse in New Zealand in 1977, and holds a bachelor's degree in nursing and certificates in stomal therapy and palliative care. She has worked as a clinical nurse consultant in surgical nursing, wound care, and stomal therapy in both acute-care and community-care settings. Jenny is a founding and life member of the Western Australian Wound Care Association. Jenny was also a founding member and treasurer of the Australian Wound Management Association (AWMA), of which she is the current president. Jenny contributed to the development of the AWMA's Clinical Practice Guidelines for the Prediction and Prevention of Pressure Ulcers. She has been the editor of *Primary Intention—the Australian Journal of Wound Management* since its inception in 1993.

Jenny is also a reviewer for the *Journal of Wound Ostomy and Continence Nursing*. She is completing a PhD at the University of Western Australia through the Faculty of Surgery and Pathology. Her thesis examines whether clinical practice guidelines for pressure ulcers reduce the prevalence of these ulcers and improve clinicians' knowledge of them. Jenny has published and presented her work in Australia, the USA, Ireland, Europe, and New Zealand.

Genevieve Sadler
Chapter 18

Dr Genevieve Sadler holds bachelor's degrees in medicine and surgery and is the surgical research registrar at Fremantle Hospital (Western Australia) where she works in the Leg Ulcer Clinic and conducts research on wound healing. Her special interest in dermatology has developed since she completed the Australasian College of Dermatologists' First Part Examination in 2002. Genevieve is studying for a master's degree in public health and is the medical representative on the Western Australian Wound Care Association Committee.

Michael Stacey
Chapter 18

Professor Michael Stacey is the head of the School of Surgery and Pathology, University of Western Australia. He is a vascular surgeon who was formerly the president of the Australian Wound Management Association and chairman of the World Union of Wound Healing Societies. Michael's research interest is in chronic venous disease and wound healing. His research work includes clinical trials and evaluation of clinical treatments for wounds, as well as basic research into the impaired healing of venous ulcers using cellular and molecular biology.

Terry Swanson
Chapter 6

Terry Swanson is a registered nurse who holds a diploma of nursing, a postgraduate certificate in perioperative nursing, and a diploma in health sciences. She is a member of the Royal College of Nursing, Australia. Terry is the clinical consultant responsible for administering wound-management services at South West Healthcare (Victoria, Australia). She has held positions of responsibility in local, state, and national wound-management professional bodies. As a member of the Australian Wound Management Association (AWMA) subcommittee, Terry participated in the development of the AWMA national 'Standards for Wound Management'. Terry has presented at local, state, national, and international conferences. She is awaiting endorsement as a Nurse Practitioner. Terry will complete her master's degree in 2005. Her thesis explores nurses' perception of the variables influencing wound management practice.

Sue Templeton

Subject specialist editor; Chapters 1, 3, 4, 10, and 11

Sue Templeton is a registered nurse who holds a bachelor's degree in nursing. She is currently undertaking a master's degree in nursing. Sue has more than 16 years' experience in the management of acute and chronic wounds, and has initiated wound-management policies, designed wound-assessment tools, and contributed to the development of a clinical pathway for the management of venous leg ulcers. Sue frequently conducts wound-management education for nurses in a variety of settings and has published and presented at local and national forums. She is currently employed as the advanced wound specialist and clinical nurse consultant with the Royal District Nursing Service of South Australia. Sue is also a clinical tutor with the University of Adelaide, a member of the South Australian Wound Management Association, the South Australian Society for Vascular Nursing, and the Australian Council of Community Nursing Services.

Carolina Weller

Chapter 2

Carolina Weller is a registered nurse and midwife who holds a bachelor's degree in nursing and a master's degree in education. She has worked in wound-care nursing for several years with interests in clinical practice, education, and research. Carolina coordinated the graduate certificate and graduate diploma of wound care at Monash University (Victoria, Australia). She is senior lecturer and coordinator of nursing studies at La Trobe University (Melbourne, Australia).

Chapter 1
On Being Wounded

Sue Templeton

Introduction

From the moment of birth and the cutting of the umbilical cord, every person is reliant on the body's healing mechanisms. From then until death, people are at the mercy of the environment and its many potential hazards. Wounding is part of everyday life. Although many people need to deal with only relatively minor cuts and scrapes, others experience major wounds.

'Every person is reliant on the body's healing mechanisms … wounding is part of everyday life.'

A wound is 'an injury to the integument or underlying structures that may or may not result in a loss of skin integrity' (Carville 2001, p. 10). Wounds can result from many causes. Trauma and accidental injuries are common causes. Some disease processes also produce wounds. Surgeons deliberately create wounds to perform operations. Indeed, in the past, wounds were deliberately created in an effort to cure various non-surgical diseases, including mental illnesses.

In many cultures, wounds are deliberately created as part of cultural or religious beliefs. And there is a growing trend in developed countries to undergo wounding to alter physical appearance to achieve 'beauty' or 'agelessness'.

Wounds often leave the person with a permanent 'reminder' in the form of a scar. But even without a physical scar, wounding and its consequences can have significant physical and psychological effects on wounded persons and those around them.

History of wound management

Wounds are common, and treatment of wounds has therefore been undertaken since prehistoric times. Cave paintings in Spain, dating from 25,000 years ago, illustrate common wounds (Bale & Jones 1997). Wound treatments varied according to cultural and religious beliefs, the level of societal development, and available resources. Blood loss and infection from traumatic wounds were major causes of death.

For thousands of years, plant-based applications have been used on wounds. Various plants and other applications have been used for their antimicrobial and astringent properties, for cleansing, and as aids to healing (Bale & Jones 1997). To stop wounds bleeding, leaves, sand, and dung have been applied. Wound cleansers have included salt water, milk, wine, and vinegar. Dressings have consisted of honey, lard, beef, or resins. Sea sponges soaked in vinegar or wine have been used to fill cavities.

Wound edges have been held together with thorns or strips of gum-soaked cloth (Baxter 2002). Early suturing involved the use of thorn needles and primitive thread. Surgery was well advanced in India in the first millennium BC. However, in other countries, surgery was seldom performed and techniques were very basic (Bale & Jones 1997).

Wars had a major influence on wound-management techniques. In early conflicts, boiling oil was often used to cauterise wounds (Wattis, Mayhew & Hillier 1997). Many of the advances in surgery and dressing techniques were developed as a result of the huge numbers of injuries sustained during war.

The twentieth century saw a number of major developments in wound management. Antisepsis and the discovery of antibiotics had a major impact on the management of infections, and dramatically improved outcomes for people with wounds.

Table 1.1 (below) lists some significant individuals and their contributions in the history of wound management.

Table 1.1 Important people in wound management
AUTHOR'S PRESENTATION ADAPTED FROM BAXTER (2002) AND BALE & JONES (1997)

Name	Era	Contribution
Hippocrates	460–379 BC	Described many diseases Promoted early haemostasis Encouraged suppuration of wounds
Celsus	25 BC–37 AD	Described the four classic signs and symptoms of inflammation—rubor (redness), calor (heat), tumor (swelling), dolor (pain) Advocated early closure of fresh wounds and debridement of contaminated wounds
Galen	129–200 AD	Promoted theory of 'laudable pus'—naturally occurring pus should be allowed to continue to discharge from the wound to aid healing; misinterpreted in the Middle Ages when wounds were deliberately contaminated to produce pus
Paracelsus	1493–1541	Proposed the theory of 'circulating juices' (which kept organs and tissues healthy) Advocated the use of minerals on wounds
Sir Charles Bell and contemporaries	early 1800s	Greater use and refinement of surgical techniques and instruments—debridement, control of haemorrhage, and surgical ligation—but many people still died of sepsis and tetanus
Louis Pasteur	1822–95	Discovered microorganisms (including bacteria) Developed heat sterilisation
Joseph Lister	1827–1912	Developed aseptic principles and applied Pasteur's sterilisation techniques to patient care Used carbolic acid as an antiseptic Improved level of cleanliness during surgery and significantly improved postoperative survival rates
Joseph Gamgee	1828–86	Promoted gentle wound-healing Developed an absorbent cotton-wool and gauze dressing
George Winter	1927–81	Undertook experiments on pigs; compared the healing rates of wounds left to dry out with those covered in an occlusive film dressing Credited with being the founder of moist wound-healing principles

Wound management continues to develop. The focus of much research is now on the physiology and pathophysiology of wound-healing with a view to an improved understanding of the healing process and how it can be influenced. New and exciting advances are being made in tissue engineering, dermal replacement, scar minimisation, and wound-management therapies. The focus of modern wound management has evolved from simply surviving wounding to the rapid restoration of form and function by overcoming barriers to healing.

Despite the advances in wound management in developed nations, some countries still struggle to provide a basic level of health care. Wars continue to ravage many parts of the globe, causing grievous injuries and death. Dressings, antibiotics, and analgesics are in short supply in many of these countries, despite the efforts of humanitarian organisations and individuals who contribute time, money, and personal effort in an effort to provide a reasonable standard of care to improve healthcare outcomes.

Nursing a person with a wound

Caring for a person with a wound provides nurses with an opportunity to establish an intimate therapeutic nursing relationship. When dressing wounds, the nurse has contact with structures of the body normally concealed by the integument. Deep wounds can expose structures (such as tendon, bone, joints, and muscles) that are usually seen only in the operating theatre.

'A wound is, in the most basic sense, a threat to a person's integrity.'

It is easy for nurses to overlook the effect that this has on a person with a wound, and on others close to the person. Nurses should be aware that it can be devastating for a person to look down and see a mangled mess of flesh, muscle, and bone. A wound is, in the most basic sense, a threat to a person's integrity. In recognising the reality of this threat, nurses must treat people with dignity and respect. Nurses should avoid thinking of the patient as 'the pressure ulcer in bed 5', or the 'really interesting abdominal wound breakdown'.

Staff members on ward rounds in hospitals are notorious for focusing attention only on the wound—rather than addressing the *person who has the wound*. Students are brought in during dressing changes to view wounds that are especially large or especially 'interesting'. In many cases, prior consent is not obtained. All of this can result in the patient feeling that he or she is an exhibit. In their role as patient advocates, nurses have a professional responsibility to encourage consideration of the whole person.

Many models have been created to explain nursing theory, nursing care, and the patient–nurse relationship. Such models can assist inexperienced wound-care nurses to construct a framework for the care they provide (Bale & Jones 1997), and can help them to understand the physical, psychological, and emotional response of patients to wounding. Whichever nursing model is chosen, the patient and his or her needs must be at the centre of the framework.

'In their role as patient advocates, nurses have a professional responsibility to encourage consideration of the whole person.'

Although the application of nursing models can be difficult in times of staff shortages and economic rationalism, there are simple strategies that nurses can employ to promote holistic care. When planning and attending to nursing care, nurses should always involve their patients. Therapeutic relationships can be developed with patients by ascertaining what is important to them. If proper consideration is given to input from both patients and healthcare professionals, realistic and appropriate goals can be set. In this way, care can be truly individualised.

The impact of wounding

There are many factors that can affect a patient's responses and behaviour. In addition to the significant physical impact of a wound, the psychological, emotional, and social effects cannot be overlooked. The story of Matt (Box, page 6) illustrates the case of a young man whose concerns went beyond the immediate physical effects of his injury.

Nurses play a pivotal role in coordinating patient management. When performing dressings, nurses have an ideal opportunity to explore patients'

Matt

Matt was a 30-year-old man who had been involved in a motor-vehicle accident. He had sustained a fracture to his right femur and a compound fracture of his right tibia and fibula. The fracture of his femur was reduced and fixed internally. Due to the multiple fractures of his tibia, external fixation was applied to stabilise the fragments.

Matt had also sustained significant soft-tissue damage. Much of the skin, subcutaneous tissue, and muscle of his right lower leg had been torn away in the accident, leaving a large wound. While Matt was waiting for plastic surgery, nurses dressed his wound regularly and frequently.

Matt expressed his distress with the injury he had sustained, and revealed that he feared for the long-term appearance and function of his leg. However, his main concerns were related to his social and family situation. Matt was married and had two small children. He was the sole income-earner and had been employed in his current job for only 18 months. He was concerned for the welfare of his family if he was unable to earn income in the future. He was also worried about how his wife was managing without him at home, and was concerned about her having to travel repeatedly to visit him in the hospital.

The nurses listened carefully to Matt's concerns. They supported him in his distress, and, with his agreement, arranged for a social worker to discuss welfare assistance and social support.

concerns and issues. Sympathetic listening and prompt referral to other healthcare professionals can help to address many social and psychological problems. With good planning and communication, a seamless transition can be achieved among organisations and levels of care. The Box on page 7 explores these issues in the context of a leg ulcer.

Patients as partners in care

Providing effective education

Patient education 'increases patients' knowledge, contributes to behavioural change and helps patients make informed decisions about their care' (Edwards, Moffatt & Franks 2002, p. 35). Different patients require varying

Living with a leg ulcer

Even when patients remain mobile, living with a chronic leg ulcer can have negative physical, psychological, and social effects (Douglas 2001). Issues that can cause anxiety for a person living with a leg ulcer include pain, wound exudate, loss of control, social isolation, reduced ability to perform activities of daily living, lack of transport, loss of self-esteem, inconvenience of dressings, and anxiety about healing prospects (Cullum & Roe 1998; Douglas 2001).

Living with a chronic leg ulcer can lead to depression, self-neglect, and lack of adherence to care regimens. Younger persons are often concerned about work performance, financial security, and mobility.

Nurses need to be alert to anxiety-related signs and symptoms. Some issues can be addressed by nurses—such as providing aids for showering or mobility, arranging for a community bus to collect the patient for shopping trips, and making links with community organisations that provide services and volunteers. Liaison with the patient's family, general practitioner, and other healthcare professionals can be beneficial.

More serious or persistent signs and symptoms might require professional assistance. Referral to a social worker, psychologist, or psychiatrist might be necessary.

In some communities, specialist leg-ulcer clinics have been established. These provide skilled comprehensive care in an environment in which many people with leg ulcers are treated concurrently. Some clinics have a room where patients can sit and have a cup of tea or coffee and socialise with others. Such clinics can provide peer support and empathy as patients develop relationships with other people living with leg ulcers (Lindsay 2001).

amounts and types of information. Some want detailed explanations, whereas others are content with minimal information.

Education involves more than merely handing out a leaflet or providing a few instructions. The most effective approach is to use a combination of educational strategies that are tailored to the patient's level of understanding and preferred method of learning. Strategies can include diagrams, pictures, leaflets, verbal instructions, and demonstrations—or a combination of these. Nurses should use simple language, avoid medical and nursing terminology, and give consistent information (Edwards, Moffatt & Franks 2002). This will promote understanding and the adoption of appropriate health behaviours.

Patients should be asked to paraphrase instructions in their own words and encouraged to ask questions. However, an absence of questions, or an ability to recite information or terminology, does not necessarily mean that patients have understood the information provided. People do not always feel empowered to ask questions, and many do not feel that they are in control of their decisions when dealing with health professionals (Lindsay 2001). A professional nursing relationship based on trust and open communication is essential to patient education and participation.

'A professional nursing relationship based on trust and open communication is essential to effective patient education and participation.'

The information that is provided should be reinforced, and opportunities should be provided for patients to discuss progress and problems. It is the responsibility of the primary treating health professional to provide sufficient information to allow a patient to make informed decisions regarding his or her care (Staunton & Chiarella 2003). In wound management the nurse often undertakes care on a regular basis. Nurses therefore have a responsibility to ensure that patients understand their conditions and the rationale for treatment. Patients also need to be informed of any other options for treatment and the consequences of declining treatment (Staunton & Chiarella 2003).

Informed decision-making and active participation can occur only when relevant and adequate information is provided, and if patients are viewed as partners in their care.

Ability to adhere to treatment regimens

There is a positive link between understanding pathophysiology and adherence to recommended treatment interventions (Edwards, Moffatt & Franks 2002). Adherence to a prescribed treatment regimen is often referred to as 'compliance' (Jones 1998). However, the terms 'adherence' and 'compliance' have different meanings.

Compliance implies that patients should do what they are told. In contrast, *adherence* implies that patients choose to follow recommendations regarding care.

There are times when the expectations and behaviours of patients do not meet the expectations and behaviours of nurses (Selim, Lewis & Templeton 2001). Nurses should avoid blaming or judging patients when they do not follow treatment regimens. Rather, nurses should try to ascertain why a patient is unable or unwilling to adhere to the recommended treatment. Reasons for non-adherence to care can include:

'Nurses should avoid blaming or judging patients when they do not follow treatment regimens.'

- a language barrier;
- poor educational techniques by health professionals;
- lack of patient confidence in the treating health professional;
- memory loss and impaired decision-making capacity;
- cultural differences;
- financial constraints; and
- physical limitations.

If the reasons for non-adherence are identified and understood, nurses are better placed to develop strategies to overcome the problems or to reach a compromise that is acceptable to a patient.

On some occasions a nurse and a patient are unable to reach a compromise. In these situations, nurses should consider the priorities of nursing care. A weekly visit—to ensure that the wound is not infected and to provide an opportunity for the patient to discuss his or her perceptions— is better than no nursing input at all.

Some patients decline all treatment. Persons of full legal capacity have a fundamental legal right to withhold consent to treatment (Staunton & Chiarella 2003). Individual legal requirements regarding consent to treatment vary among jurisdictions, and nurses should be familiar with the legal requirements in their own areas of practice. In general, if a patient declines any nursing treatment, a nurse should make every reasonable effort to inform the patient of the possible consequences of no nursing care. The conversation and the patient's response should be clearly and carefully documented. All other healthcare professionals involved in the patient's care should be informed that the patient has declined treatment.

Promoting optimal wound-management practice

Barriers to evidence-based practice

Wound management is no longer based on tradition and superstition. Modern wound management is based on scientific principles and research. In recent years, wound management has become a specialty area of practice for nurses, doctors, and other healthcare professionals.

However, in some areas, individuals adhere to traditional practices based on personal preference and outdated beliefs. Nurses can be faced with requests to use solutions, dressings, and techniques that are not based on evidence; in some cases they can even be contraindicated by evidence. Nurses are accountable for providing high-quality, evidence-based care that promotes optimal health for patients (RCNA 2000). By following outdated or potentially harmful practices, nurses are failing in their professional responsibility to their patients. However, nurses often feel powerless and frustrated in their desire to implement evidence-based practices that will improve wound outcomes.

'Nurses can be faced with requests that are not based on evidence; in some cases they can even be contraindicated by evidence.'

Resistance to changing practices can occur for various reasons— including perceived threats to self-interest, erroneous perceptions, and fear of losing something valuable (Wattis, Mayhew & Hillier 1997).

There are numerous strategies that can produce positive changes in wound management. These include (Wattis Mayhew & Hillier 1997):

- bedside teaching;
- formal and informal lectures using peer speakers;

- wound-management courses;
- seminars, conferences, and workshops;
- demonstration of techniques;
- presentation of new products;
- discussion groups;
- distribution of journal articles and texts; and
- implementation of policies and guidelines.

Complementary therapies

Complementary therapies are becoming more prominent in health care. Nurses are often asked for their opinion on complementary therapies. In providing a response, nurses should be guided by relevant legal, professional, and ethical guidelines, and by their own professional experience and personal beliefs.

'The achievement of optimal outcomes for patients is always paramount.'

Nurses must consider the effect that their advice could have on their patients. The achievement of optimal outcomes for patients is always paramount.

Legal aspects and professional conduct

Most legal claims against healthcare professionals are founded on allegations of negligence. Patients or their relatives can seek financial compensation for past, present, and future pain, for physical and psychological harm, and for financial loss. These might be due to acts of commission or acts of omission (Staunton & Chiarella 2003).

In many jurisdictions, negligence is founded on four general legal principles. For negligence to have occurred, all of the four criteria must be met (on the balance of probabilities). The Box on page 12 summarises these legal conditions.

The development of pressure ulcers is one area of wound management in which litigation is common in the United States and the United Kingdom. Despite staff shortages, financial constraints, and

Legal basis for negligence

In many jurisdictions, negligence is founded on four general legal principles. For negligence to have occurred, all of the following four criteria must be met (on the balance of probabilities).

1. Duty of care
The nurse must have owed the patient a *duty of care*. In establishing a legal duty of care, the *expected standard of care* must also be established.

2. Care below expected standard
On the occasion in question, the nurse's care must have *fallen below the expected standard*. A breach of the duty of care can therefore be said to have occurred.

3. Direct harm
The breach of the duty of care must have *directly resulted in harm to the patient*.

4. Reasonably foreseeable consequence
The harm caused to the patient must have been a *reasonably foreseeable consequence* of the nurse's breach of the duty of care.

ADAPTED FROM STAUNTON & CHIARELLA (2003)

increasing patient acuity, nurses have a duty of care to meet professional and organisational standards. If nurses are aware of, and active in, professional wound-management bodies, this can put political pressure on healthcare organisations to implement evidence-based standards and guidelines.

In many jurisdictions, nursing regulatory bodies can investigate accusations of inappropriate or unprofessional conduct. In many cases, these involve instances in which harm has not actually occurred, but in which the nurse's behaviour is alleged to breach legal or professional standards. If continued, such conduct might cause harm to patients, colleagues, or the nurse involved.

The influence of the trade

The treatment of wounds has become a major industry. In many countries it is a multi-million dollar business in which companies compete for a share of a very competitive market. Many treatments are marketed for wound management—including dressings, skin substitutes, sutures, lasers, whirlpools, and hyperbaric chambers.

'Nurses should seek evidence from independent, research-based literature to assess claims about products or treatments.'

Company representatives provide a valuable service in supplying product information and wound-care advice to healthcare professionals. Many companies also offer wound-education sessions. The provision of such education and information by companies is governed by documented organisational guidelines that promote consistency and transparency. However, nurses should always be aware that companies are attempting to sell their products, and nurses should therefore seek evidence from independent, research-based literature if they are to have a sound basis on which to assess claims about products or treatments.

Conclusion

Nursing a person with a wound can be a challenging and rewarding endeavour. There are many factors to be considered if nurses are to provide holistic, evidence-based care that will achieve optimal outcomes for their patients.

Nurses should always be aware that wound management encompasses physical, psychological, emotional, and social dimensions. Wound-management nurses must be skilled in the provision of the technical aspects of care. But they

'Nurses should value the personal qualities, individual characteristics, and contributions of the person living with a wound.'

should also value the personal qualities, individual characteristics, and contributions of the *person* living with a wound.

Chapter 2
The Skin and Healing
Carolina Weller

Introduction

The skin is a large, complex organ that is exposed to injury, infection, and other disease processes. Many factors affect the health of the skin—including age, nutrition, hygiene, circulation, immunity, genetic traits, psychological states, and drugs. All of these factors affect wound healing.

This chapter considers the anatomy and physiology of the skin, and how these factors affect the normal process of wound healing.

Normal skin

Structure of skin

The skin is the largest organ in the body. In adults, the skin has an area of approximately 2 square metres. Like all organs, the skin consists of various tissues that work in combination to perform certain activities.

Structurally, the skin consists of two principal parts (see Figure 2.1, page 21):

- the *epidermis*—an outer, thinner part consisting of epithelial tissue (and an external layer of keratin); and
- the *dermis*—an inner, thicker portion consisting of connective tissue (collagen and elastic fibres) and blood vessels.

Framework of the chapter

This chapter discusses the basic principles of skin and healing under the following headings.

Normal skin
- structure of skin
- functions of skin
- effects of ageing

Wounds
- definition
- classification of wounds
- acute and chronic wounds

Healing
- modes of healing
- process of wound healing
- principles of wound management
- moist wound healing
- factors that impair healing

Beneath the dermis is a subcutaneous layer—also called the *hypodermis*—which attaches the skin to underlying structures. This subcutaneous layer consists of adipose tissue and areolar tissue.

Epidermis

The epidermis is avascular and is composed of keratinised stratified squamous epithelium. This contains four types of cells.

- *Keratinocytes* are formed in the basal layers of the epidermis before migrating to the surface. As the cells move upwards they accumulate keratin—a protein that helps protect the skin and underlying tissues.

- *Melanocytes* produce melanin—a pigment responsible for skin colour and absorbing ultraviolet (UV) radiation.

- *Langerhans' cells* play a role in immune responses and are easily damaged by UV radiation.
- *Merkel cells* are located in the deepest layer of the epidermis of hairless skin. These cells are thought to play a part in touch sensation.

The epidermis consists of distinct layers. In most regions of the body, there are four recognisable layers. Where exposure to friction is greatest (such as in the palms and soles), the epidermis is thicker (1–2 mm) and five layers can be identified.

Constant exposure of skin to friction or pressure stimulates the formation of callus.

Dermis

The dermis is composed of connective tissue—collagen and elastic fibres. The few cells in the dermis include fibroblasts, macrophages, and adipocytes. The combination of collagen and elastic fibres provides strength, extensibility, and elasticity. Small tears in the skin due to extensive stretching remain visible as silver-white streaks called striae.

The dermis consists of two layers. The superficial layer is called the *papillary* layer. It consists of areolar connective tissue and small, finger-like projections called dermal papillae. Dermal papillae cause ridges in the epidermis, which produce fingerprints and help people to grip objects. With age the dermal papillae flatten, and this is a contributing factor to shear injuries in older persons.

The deeper layer of the dermis is called the *reticular* layer. It consists of dense, irregular connective tissue, adipose tissue, hair follicles, nerves, and sebaceous (oil) glands. It is attached to underlying bone and muscle by the subcutaneous layer.

Functions of skin

There are many different functions of the skin. In terms of wound healing, five functions are especially important. These are:

- protection;
- sensation;

- regulation of body temperature;
- excretion; and
- synthesis of vitamin D.

These are described in more detail in the Box below.

Functions of the skin

In terms of wound healing, five functions of the skin are especially important.

Protection

The skin covers the body and provides a physical barrier that protects underlying tissues from physical abrasion, bacterial invasion, dehydration, and UV radiation.

Sensation

The skin contains many nerve endings and receptors that react to stimuli and produce sensations such as touch, pressure, heat, and pain.

Regulation of body temperature

The skin plays three main roles in regulation of body temperature:

- in response to high temperature or strenuous exercise, the evaporation of sweat from the surface of the skin lowers body temperature;
- the circulatory mechanisms of vasodilatation and vasoconstriction control blood flow to the skin, thus regulating heat loss; and
- adipose tissue and hair provide insulation to the skin.

Excretion

Small amounts of water, salts, and organic compounds are excreted by the sweat glands.

Synthesis of vitamin D

Exposure of the skin to UV radiation helps to produce vitamin D—which assists in the absorption of calcium and phosphorus from the digestive system.

Effects of ageing

Ageing decreases the efficiency of wound healing. The skin is constantly ageing, but pronounced changes do not become apparent until a person's age approaches 50 years. With increased age, cell division and replication slows down, re-epithelialisation is less efficient, and the hair and nails grow more slowly.

'Ageing skin is more prone to wounding—and heals more slowly when a wound does occur.'

Collagen fibres decrease in number, become brittle, and lose their organised structure. Elastic fibres lose some elasticity, thicken into clumps, and fray. As a result of these changes, the skin forms indentations ('wrinkles').

Fibroblasts, which produce collagen and elastic fibres, decrease in number, and macrophages become less efficient.

The number of Langerhans' cells decreases—thus diminishing the immune response of the skin. The sebaceous glands function less effectively, and this leads to dry and broken skin that is more susceptible to infection. Production of sweat also diminishes.

There is a decrease in the number of normally functioning melanocytes. This causes grey hair and atypical skin pigmentation. An increase in the size of some melanocytes produces blotching.

Aged skin heals poorly and becomes more susceptible to pathological conditions such as pruritic dermatitis, pressure ulcers, and cancer.

For all of these reasons, ageing skin is more prone to wounding— and heals more slowly when a wound does occur.

Wounds

Definition

A wound can be defined as any interruption to the integrity of tissue. A wound can affect the skin, mucosa, or internal organs.

Classification of wounds

Descriptive classification

Skin wounds can be classified descriptively by the layers involved. A commonly used classification is to describe wounds that involve only the epidermis as 'superficial' wounds. If the wound involves the dermis, this is described as a 'partial-thickness' wound. 'Full-thickness' wounds reach into the subcutaneous tissue (or deeper); they can also involve muscle, tendon, or bone.

Wound staging

In addition to the descriptive classification (above), wounds can also be classified in stages. The classification (as shown schematically in Figure 2.1, page 21) is in four stages.

- *Stage 1:* The superficial layers of the epidermis are intact, but there is persistent (non-blanchable) erythema or discolouration.
- *Stage 2:* There is loss of skin integrity, with damage to the epidermal and dermal layers of the skin. There can also be erythema of surrounding tissues and low-to-moderate exudate.
- *Stage 3:* There is loss of subcutaneous tissue with cavity formation. There is often a moderate-to-high level of exudate.
- *Stage 4:* There is a loss of subcutaneous tissue with a cavity formation involving muscle, tendon, and/or bone. A high level of exudate is common at this stage.

Acute and chronic wounds

Wounds can also be classified as *acute* or *chronic*. This refers to the time taken for a wound to heal.

Acute wounds progress through a predictable series of events that result in a healed wound. (For more on normal healing, see 'Healing', page 22.)

In contrast, *chronic* wounds fail to proceed through an orderly and timely healing process. A wound is considered to be chronic when it does not follow the normal healing pattern in an expected timeframe. Most wounds heal in 4–6 weeks, and a wound that does not heal in this time can be considered 'chronic'. Many wounds seen in clinical practice are chronic in nature, and the management of chronic wounds can be difficult. In some instances, chronic wounds never heal. The most common locations for

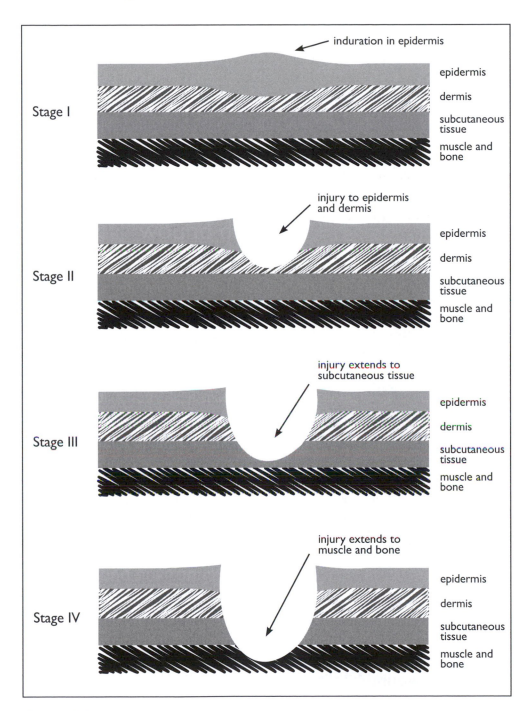

Figure 2.1 Wound staging
AUTHOR'S SCHEMATIC PRESENTATION (ADAPTED FROM HARDING 2001)

chronic wounds are the lower legs and feet, and over bony prominences (such as the hips, heels and sacral region).

Healing

Modes of healing

Traditionally, healing of wounds has been classified as healing by 'primary intention' or healing by 'secondary intention'. The Box below provides more information. Figure 2.2 (page 23) provides a schematic indication of these modes of healing.

Modes of healing

Healing by primary intention

In healing by *primary intention* there is minimal tissue loss. Wound edges are closely approximated with sutures, clips, tape, or tissue glue. 'Delayed primary intention' is said to occur when healing by primary intention is delayed for 3–5 days by infection, foreign bodies, or a requirement for debridement. In healing by primary intention, scarring is either absent or minimal.

Healing by secondary intention

In healing by *secondary intention*, wound healing is delayed. It progresses through granulation, contraction, and epithelialisation. In healing by secondary intention, scarring is usually evident.

Wound healing can also be achieved by skin grafts or flaps. These surgical techniques are usually undertaken if a surgeon feels that healing by primary intention or secondary intention is impossible or undesirable.

Process of wound healing

The wound-healing process begins with haemostasis (control of bleeding). Platelets are activated when exposed to extravascular collagen. Platelet adhesion to collagen activates them to release growth factors and

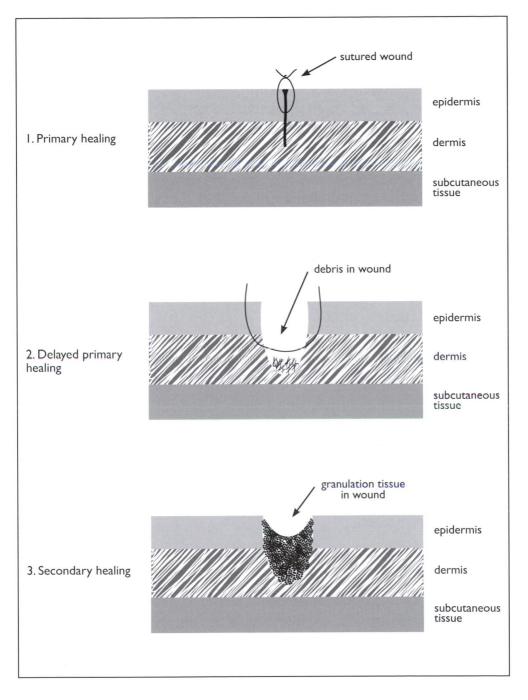

Figure 2.2 Modes of healing

AUTHOR'S SCHEMATIC PRESENTATION (ADAPTED FROM CARVILLE 2001)

adhesive glycoproteins. This makes the platelets 'sticky'. Meanwhile, enzymes of the 'clotting cascade' convert fibrinogen to fibrin. The fibrin molecules and aggregated platelets provide the bulk of a 'clot'. (Tortora 1997).

Haemostasis is followed by the *three phases of healing*:

- inflammation;
- proliferation; and
- maturation.

These phases overlap and merge together in a continuous process.

Inflammatory phase

The inflammatory phase lasts about 72 hours. This phase prepares the injured site for rebuilding of new tissue. The inflammatory response is initiated by the release of chemical mediators and growth factors from damaged cells and platelets.

Leucocytes are attracted to the wound site by these chemical mediators. Within six hours neutrophils begin to destroy and remove cellular debris, bacteria, and foreign bodies at the wound site.

Monocytes move into the wound site with neutrophils. These monocytes later differentiate into macrophages. In a sterile wound, neutrophils begin to disappear after 72 hours, leaving macrophages as the most common type of cells. Macrophages continue wound debridement, attract fibroblasts, and secrete proteases, growth factors, and leukotrienes. These biologically active substances ensure ongoing progress of the wound-healing process.

Proliferative phase

The proliferative phase includes angiogenesis (formation of new blood vessels), contraction of the wound, and re-epithelialisation of the wound.

During angiogenesis, capillary 'buds' are formed. These link up with the existing capillary network to provide essential oxygen and nutrients. New collagen is formed, and this cross-links with elastin and the new vascular base to form the collagen matrix. The result is granulation tissue.

The tissues and skin surrounding the wound are mobilised and pulled together. This contraction decreases the size of the defect.

Phases of healing

This portion of the text discusses the three phases of healing:

- inflammation;
- proliferation; and
- maturation.

   These phases overlap and merge together in a continuous process. They are described in more detail in the text.

While these changes are occurring in the wound, the epithelium is being restored at the wound surface. Re-epithelialisation of the wound begins within a couple of hours of the injury. Some epithelial cells come from the wound edge, whereas others arise from epithelial appendages within the wound bed. These epithelial cells migrate under the scab and over the underlying connective tissue.

Maturation phase

During the maturation phase (sometimes called the 'remodelling phase'), the collagen fibres within the wound are realigned and strengthened—thus increasing the tensile strength of the wound.

In wound-healing by *secondary intention*, complete coverage by epithelial tissue can take a long time—depending on various factors that affect healing. In some cases of healing by secondary intention, complete healing and maturation can take 12–18 months.

Principles of wound management

Wound management involves caring for the *person* with a wound—not just the wound itself. Person-centred nursing care considers the physical, psychological, social, economic, and spiritual dimensions of care— beginning with a comprehensive patient assessment. (Assessment is discussed in greater detail in Chapter 3, 'Assessment and Documentation', page 33.)

Following a comprehensive assessment, wound care should follow the principles of wound management:

- identify wound aetiology (cause);
- identify and control factors that impair healing;
- set long-term and short-term objectives;
- implement a management regimen;
- review and revise the management plan frequently; and
- plan for maintenance of healed tissue and/or quality of life.

Identify wound aetiology (cause)

Identification of the cause of a wound provides information about the likely pathophysiology of the wound and assists in planning an appropriate management regimen. Possible causes include: pressure, circulatory insufficiency, and burns.

Identify and control factors that impair healing

There are many factors that can impair healing. Not all of these can be controlled or eliminated. Identification of factors that can impair healing assists in assessing the healing potential of a wound, the planning of long-term objectives, and setting timeframes for wound progress.

Set long-term and short-term objectives

Realistic, measurable objectives should be identified and documented. The long-term objective of wound management is healing of the wound or, if this is not possible, a satisfactory outcome for the quality of life of the patient. Short-term objectives refer to factors that need to be managed in the immediate future with a view to achieving the long-term objectives.

'Realistic, measurable objectives should be identified and documented.'

Implement a management regimen

A management regimen is based on an assessment of wound aetiology and identified objectives. Interventions should be individually tailored to meet the needs of the wound and the patient. These can include appropriate

Principles of wound management

This portion of the text discusses the principles of wound healing:
- identify wound aetiology (cause);
- identify and control factors that impair healing;
- set long-term and short-term objectives;
- implement a management regimen;
- review and revise the management plan frequently; and
- plan for maintenance of healed tissue and/or maintenance of quality of life.

dressings, nutritional interventions, use of pressure-reducing devices, compression therapy, and lifestyle changes.

Review and revise the management plan frequently

Re-evaluation and revision of short-term objectives should be carried out at least once a month—in conjunction with a systematic, documented wound assessment. If a wound with healing potential has not responded to the current management regimen in one month, a comprehensive reassessment should be undertaken (going back to reassessment of aetiology, and proceeding through all principles again).

Plan for maintenance of healed tissue and/or quality of life

It is important to educate patients on how to manage their healed wounds. If applicable, this includes education on preventing recurrence. For people with limited healing potential, strategies should be implemented to optimise quality of life while living with a wound.

Moist wound healing

Modern wound management involves moist wound healing. This has been shown to be significantly more effective than the dry-healing techniques of the past.

Fragile epithelial cells migrate more freely and remain viable longer in a wound that is not dehydrated or covered by scab formation

(Winter 1962). Epithelialisation of a wound therefore occurs more quickly if a moist wound-healing environment is maintained.

Wound exudate contains growth factors and nutrients, and has antimicrobial properties. Exudate significantly increases the rate of healing.

Factors that impair healing

Nurses need to be aware of factors that can impair wound healing. These factors fall into two categories—*intrinsic factors* (factors related to the patient) and *extrinsic factors* (external factors affecting healing). These are listed in the Box below.

Factors that impair healing

Factors that impair wound healing fall into two categories—*intrinsic factors* (factors related to the patient) and *extrinsic factors* (external factors affecting healing). The factors listed below are discussed in more detail in the text.

Intrinsic factors
Intrinsic factors include:
- health status;
- age;
- body build;
- lifestyle factors; and
- nutritional status.

Extrinsic factors
Extrinsic factors include:
- mechanical stress;
- debris;
- temperature;
- desiccation or maceration;
- infection; and
- chemical stress.

Intrinsic factors

Health status

Certain factors in general health status can affect wound healing. These include such factors as cardiovascular disease, arteriosclerosis; peripheral vascular disease, metabolic disorders (such as diabetes), inflammatory disorders, malabsorption syndromes, anaemia, immune disorders, cancer, and immobility.

Age

As previously discussed (see this chapter, page 19), healing is slower in older people because metabolism is slower, skin is thinner and less elastic, and peripheral blood flow is decreased.

Body build

Both obesity and debilitation can adversely affect wound healing.

Obesity is associated with immobility, diminished peripheral blood flow, increased risk of wound dehiscence (opening and gaping), hernia formation, and trapping of moisture in skin folds.

Thin and debilitated people lack energy stores to maintain metabolic processes.

Lifestyle factors

Smoking decreases peripheral blood flow and oxygen-carrying capacity. Alcohol abuse can result in liver disease and digestive disorders that can lead to malnutrition and anaemia. Stress and anxiety increase glucocorticoid release.

Nutritional status

Wound healing requires extra intake of protein, calories, vitamins, and minerals. Essential minerals include zinc, copper, and iron. Vitamins A, C, and B complex are required. Adequate fluid intake is required to maintain cellular hydration. (Nutrition and healing is discussed in more detail in Chapter 7, 'Nutrition and Healing', page 105.)

Extrinsic factors

Mechanical stress

Mechanical stress can create a wound or disrupt the healing of an existing wound. Such mechanical forces can include pressure, friction, and shearing forces.

Debris

Debris includes necrotic tissue, scabs, excess slough, fibres, and suture fragments. Such debris impairs epithelial migration and supply of nutrients. Foreign bodies prolong the inflammatory phase and increase the risk of infection.

Temperature

A temperature of 37 degrees Celsius is optimal for mitotic activity. Temperature extremes cause tissue damage. Dressing changes can cause a significant drop in temperature.

Desiccation or maceration

Both excessive dryness and excessive moisture can adversely affect wound healing.

Desiccation (dryness) causes cell death and forms a physical barrier to the migration of epithelial cells from the wound edges.

Maceration (excessive moisture) can be caused by excessive exudate, perspiration, or urine and faeces. Maceration weakens the wound edges and predisposes the wound to infection

Infection

Infection slows wound healing by release of bacterial toxins that affect fibroblast activity and prolong the inflammatory phase.

Clinical signs of infection include erythema, oedema, tenderness, elevated temperature, induration, purulent exudate, and malodour.

Swabs can be taken for microscopy and culture, but a wound biopsy is the 'gold standard' of diagnosis.

Treatment consists of antibiotics (local and/or systemic). Topical antiseptics have limited usefulness.

Chemical stress

Some topical antiseptics are cytotoxic, and can damage healing tissue.

Conclusion

Understanding the anatomy and physiology of skin, and the types and phases of healing, assists nurses to make informed decisions about how they manage people with wounds. Several intrinsic and extrinsic factors can impair wound healing.

Nurses need to consider the whole picture—including the aetiology of the wound and factors that can affect healing. Effective wound-care nursing requires an awareness of caring for patients as persons—rather than dealing with a wound in isolation.

'Effective wound-care nursing requires an awareness of caring for patients as persons— rather than dealing with a wound in isolation.'

Chapter 3

Assessment and Documentation

Sue Templeton

Introduction

The cornerstones of wound management are sound assessment and accurate documentation (Banks 1998). If nurses are to plan and deliver high-quality care, they require knowledge of the factors that affect wound healing and an understanding of the common terminology associated with wound characteristics. Training in assessment methods and the use of consistent terminology facilitates reliable documentation and communication.

'The cornerstones of wound management are sound assessment and accurate documentation.'

Principles of wound management

The principles of effective wound management are based on a comprehensive assessment and the development of a wound-management regimen tailored to the person's individual needs. Consideration should be given to the person's general status (health, social, economic, and psychological) and to the characteristics of the wound (Morison et al. 1997).

The principles of wound management are as follows (Fergusson & MacLellan 1997).

- *Step 1:* Determine the aetiology (cause) of the wound.
- *Step 2:* Identify and eliminate (or control) any factors that might impair healing.
- *Step 3:* Determine realistic and achievable long-term and short-term objectives.
- *Step 4:* Implement an appropriate management regimen.
- *Step 5:* Monitor the response to the management regimen regularly and frequently (and reassess as necessary).
- *Step 6:* Ensure that an optimal outcome is achieved.

  Step 6 is achieved by applying the following principles.
- If the wound heals, maintain healed tissue.
- If healing is the goal of management and the wound fails to heal or progress, go back to Step 1 and reassess.
- If healing is not the goal of management (as might be the case, for example, with a malignant wound) ensure that quality of life is optimised.

Factors impairing healing

Wound assessment begins with a comprehensive assessment of the person with the wound. In carrying out their assessment, nurses should be aware of certain factors that might impair healing—and should document whether these factors are present or absent. These factors can be classified as *intrinsic* factors or *extrinsic* factors (AWMA 2002). The Box on page 35 lists some of the more important intrinsic and extrinsic factors that can impair wound healing.

'Wound assessment begins with a comprehensive assessment of the person with the wound.'

Nurses should record all information in a systematic and standardised manner. This ensures that all health professionals who are caring for the person can access relevant information on which to base an appropriate management plan (Williams 1997).

Factors impairing wound healing

Nurses should be aware of certain factors that might impair healing. As part of a comprehensive assessment, they should document whether these factors are present or absent.

Intrinsic factors

- increasing age
- poor mobility
- moisture (for example, incontinence)
- obesity
- poor nutrition
- reduced sensation
- diabetes
- liver failure
- rheumatoid arthritis
- anaemia and blood dyscrasias
- inflammatory bowel disease
- autoimmune disorders
- reduced circulation
- corticosteroid medication
- non-steroidal anti-inflammatory drugs (NSAIDs)
- cytotoxic medication
- radiotherapy

Extrinsic factors

- excessive wound exudate
- high bacterial load or infection
- wound desiccation (dryness)
- cooling of wounds below 37 degrees Celsius
- slough or necrotic tissue
- recurrent trauma
- pressure, shear, and friction
- foreign bodies
- haematoma
- local hypoxia

ADAPTED FROM CARVILLE (2001); BALE & JONES (1997); BENBOW (2002)

It is important that the long-term and short-term goals of wound management are clearly articulated. The wound-management plan is developed from these goals. The long-term goals and wound-management strategies for an elderly woman who has developed a malignant wound due to recurrence of breast cancer will be quite different from those for a young man with no significant health problems who has undergone excision of a pilonidal sinus.

'It is important that the long-term and short-term goals of wound management are clearly articulated.'

Old dressings

Assessment of old wound dressings is often overlooked. Old dressings can reveal vital information about the characteristic of the wound and the appropriateness of the dressing products that have previously been chosen.

Old dressings provide information about the amount, colour, and consistency of wound exudate. They also reveal vital information about the appropriateness of the dressing.

To facilitate moist wound healing, dressings should not adhere to the wound. Removal of adhered dressings can damage fragile granulation tissue. Leakage of exudate from dressings should also be avoided if possible. A moist tract provides a ready portal of entry for microorganisms. If dressing adhesion or leaking occurs, consideration should be given to changing the application technique, the dressing product itself, or the frequency of dressing changes.

In some instances, the old dressing can reveal information that might not be obtained from examination of the wound alone. For example, the presence of *Pseudomonas aeruginosa* can leave a characteristic fluorescent-green colouring on the old dressing that might not be present on the surface of the wound itself.

Methods of wound assessment

Regular and frequent assessment and documentation of wound characteristics allow nurses to ascertain whether the management regimen is appropriate and whether it is meeting expected outcomes (Bachand & McNichols 1999). Careful assessment and accurate documentation yield information that can be readily interpreted and easily compared with previous assessments.

Wound assessment and documentation methods include (Adderley & Nelson 2000):

- written records;
- tracings;
- photography;
- castings; and
- technological techniques.

The most common forms of wound documentation are written records, tracings, and photography. These are discussed below.

Written documentation

Written documentation of wound management is usually undertaken as part of the person's clinical record. As with other aspects of the clinical record, written reports of wound management provide an account of the treatment delivered and the person's progress. Written reports can also be used for education, research, quality control, and legal evidence (Staunton & Chiarella 2003). The recording of the person's health history, wound characteristics, and response to management thus fulfils a nurse's clinical, professional, and legal responsibilities.

'The recording of the person's health history, wound characteristics, and response to management fulfils a nurse's clinical, professional, and legal responsibilities.'

Wound-related entries can form part of the general written record or they can be documented on specialised charts or forms. Written reports should be accurate, brief, complete, legible, and objective (Staunton & Chiarella 2003). The use of phrases such as 'dressing attended' in a person's record is not useful unless such phrases are accompanied by more detailed information regarding the characteristics and progress of the wound (Williams 1997).

A wound-assessment chart is a useful tool to ensure that all wound characteristics are assessed and documented (Williams 1997). A well-designed wound-assessment chart allows easy comparison of wound characteristics over time, and thus assists nurses to determine wound progress. In addition, such charts are of assistance to nurses who are inexperienced in wound management (Bachand & McNichols 1999). A chart with prompts for each wound characteristic thus ensures that all necessary information is collected and also serves as a learning tool for inexperienced nurses.

When introducing a wound-assessment chart, training and guidelines are necessary. This ensures that nurses and other health professionals have a clear understanding of the terminology used—thus facilitating a high level of reliability in documentation. (For more on the introduction of such charts, see 'Introduction of a wound-assessment chart', this chapter, page 48.)

Tracings

To create a wound tracing, clear plastic sheeting is placed over the wound. The wound margins are then traced on the plastic with a marker pen. This is a recommended technique that provides accurate representation of wound area and shape. However, it does depend on consistent precise recording of the location of the wound margins.

Photography

Photographing wounds can be a valuable adjunct to written documentation. Photographs allow more specific identification of wound characteristics than a written record alone (Swann 2000). Photographs taken over a period of time can clearly demonstrate the progress of a wound.

'Photographing wounds can be a valuable adjunct to written documentation.'

A single-lens reflex (SLR) camera that uses 35-mm film or a digital still camera of at least 3.2-megapixel resolution should be used. A manual flash is preferable. An instant picture camera is convenient—however, it is not possible to make copies of the photographs, and some do not allow clear close-ups (Swann 2000).

Consent should be obtained from the person before taking photographs. This is especially important if the photographs might be used for purposes other than contributing to the person's clinical record (for example, for research, education, or publication). A written consent form for photography is recommended because it provides an enduring legal record.

'Consent should be obtained from the person before taking photographs … a written consent form for photography is recommended.'

Good lighting results in more accurate colour reproduction. The flash should always be used. Fluorescent lighting can alter the reproduction of colour. A plain-coloured cloth (for example, grey, blue, or green) should be used to provide a background behind the wound (Adderley & Nelson 2000). The use of white, reflective, or 'busy' backgrounds should be avoided because these can affect the quality of the photographs.

At least two photographs should be taken—one from a distance illustrating the entire body area, and one from close range to illustrate wound detail. The longer-distance photograph allows an overall perspective of the location of the wound (see Figure 3.1, page 40). When taking close-up photographs, a scale such as a disposable ruler should be placed next to the wound to provide an indication of size (see Figure 3.2, page 40).

The camera lens should be held perpendicular to the wound. If the camera lens is angled at less than 90 degrees, the appearance of the wound can be distorted (Samad et al. 2002).

Each photograph should be labelled clearly with the person's details and wound location. Confidentiality of photographs should be respected—as with other components of the person's record. Photographic prints or digital images should be stored securely to protect the rights of the person and the organisation.

Specific computer programs are available to provide nurses with quantitative wound data. These programs analyse a digital photograph to determine accurate wound size and tissue types. The person's treatment and response to interventions can also be recorded in the computer program (Santamaria, Austin & Clayton 2002).

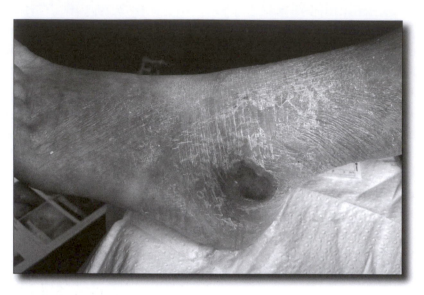

Figure 3.1 Photograph of ankle ulcer showing position of the wound
REPRODUCED WITH PERMISSION OF RDNS SA INC.

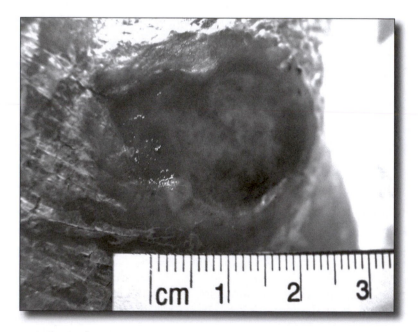

Figure 3.2 Close-up view of same ankle ulcer as shown in Figure 3.1, with rule to indicate size
REPRODUCED WITH PERMISSION OF RDNS SA INC.

Digital photographs can be emailed between health professionals. This can assist greatly in multidisciplinary management of the person. In rural and remote areas, digital photographs can be sent via email to medical specialists in large cities. Diagnosis, treatment recommendations, and monitoring of progress can all be facilitated by reducing the need for the person with a wound to travel to a medical specialist. Teleconferencing can also be used to manage persons with a wound (Samad et al. 2002).

Wound characteristics

When assessing the wound itself, there are several specific characteristics to consider. These should be evaluated at each dressing change and compared with the previous documented assessment (Bachand & McNichols 1999).

Although each characteristic should be assessed individually, the best assessment of wound status is provided by the overall clinical picture—achieved through the integration of *all* characteristics.

Through comparison of such assessments over time, nurses are able to determine wound progress.

The characteristics that should be noted include:

- wound size;
- depth or stage;
- tissue types;
- exudate;
- odour;
- surrounding skin; and
- skin eruptions.

Each of these is discussed below.

Wound size

Regular and frequent assessment of wound size is important in assessing wound progress (Goldman & Salcido 2002). A decrease in the area of a wound is an objective measurement of healing (Samad et al. 2002).

Wound size can be ascertained in various ways. There are advantages and disadvantages to each (see Table 3.1, below).

Table 3.1 Determination of wound size
AUTHOR'S PRESENTATION (ADAPTED FROM GOLDMAN & SALCIDO 2002; LANGEMO ET AL. 1998; PUDNER 2002); REPRODUCED WITH PERMISSION OF RDNS SA INC.

Method	Description	Comments
Linear measurement	Measurement of the greatest length and greatest width (width is measured perpendicular to the length)	Assumes a wound is rectangular or elliptical; might be inaccurate for irregularly shaped wounds
Wound tracing	Clear plastic sheeting is placed over the wound; wound margins are then traced on the plastic with a marker pen	Recommended technique; provides accurate representation of wound area and shape; however, does depend on consistent precise location of wound margins
Area measurement	(i) Length is multiplied by width (ii) Wound tracing is transposed onto a grid with 0.5-cm squares; the number of whole squares within the tracing is then counted to calculate the area (iii) Computer program analyses a digital photograph to determine wound area	(i) Inaccurate for irregularly shaped wounds (ii) Standardised technique is important; only full squares should be counted (not partial squares); varying the location of the grid in relation to the tracing can lead to a difference of up to 5 squares (iii) Requires specialised equipment and training; initial outlay costly; very accurate
Depth measurement	Maximum depth of the wound is measured with a sterile probe and documented	Varying depths within a wound can cause inaccuracy; does not indicate wound volume

If there are any sinus tracts or undermining, these should be noted and documented. Undermining can be represented on a wound tracing as a broken line (Bale & Jones 1997). An alternative method of documenting undermining and sinuses is to use a clockface diagram (Carville 2001)— for example: '4-cm deep sinus at 3 o'clock' or '2-cm undermining from 12 o'clock to 4 o'clock'.

Wound characteristics

When assessing the wound itself, there are several specific characteristics to consider. The characteristics that should be noted include:

- wound size;
- depth or stage;
- tissue types;
- exudate;
- odour;
- surrounding skin; and
- skin eruptions.

Each of these is discussed in detail in this part of the chapter.

Depth or stage

Wounds can be classified according to the depth of tissue injury. This provides nurses with an indication of the structures involved in the wound.

Although this staging system is widely used for describing *pressure ulcers*, it is useful for grading *most wounds* and should be used more widely (see Table 3.2, page 44).

Tissue types

The type of tissue within a wound should be noted. Unhealthy, devitalised, or necrotic tissue should usually be removed to facilitate healing and to reduce the risk of infection (Bale & Jones 1997).

The most common tissue types are (adapted from Carville 2001):

- *necrotic tissue*—black, grey, or dark blue; dead tissue that can be moist or dry;
- *slough*—yellow or whitish; devitalised tissue that can be densely adherent, soft, stringy, or spongy;
- *granulation tissue*—healthy red tissue;

Table 3.2 Staging of wounds

AUTHOR'S PRESENTATION (ADAPTED FROM AWMA 2001)

Stage	Summary	Comments
Stage 1	Non-blanchable erythema of intact skin	In dark-skinned persons the area can appear bluish or purple
Stage 2	A partial-thickness wound	Tissue loss extends through the epidermis and can involve the dermis Wound presents as a blister, abrasion, or shallow crater Wound does not extend into the subcutaneous tissue
Stage 3	A full-thickness wound	Tissue loss extends into the subcutaneous tissue and can involve undermining Wound can present as a deep crater Wound does not extend through the deep fascia
Stage 4	A full-thickness wound that extends through the deep fascia	Bone, tendon, joints, and extensive muscle destruction Sinus formation and deep cavities can be present

- *hypergranulation tissue*—an overgrowth of granulation tissue that often protrudes beyond the wound bed; red in colour with a soft, spongy, or jelly-like appearance; bleeds easily when rubbed; can delay wound healing and can force wound edges apart (Dunford 1999); and

- *epithelialising tissue*—pink tissue evident as epithelium covering the wound.

Wounds can be simply classified according to colour as 'black', 'yellow', 'red', or 'pink'. However, because many wounds contain more than one type of tissue, it is more accurate to document each tissue type as a percentage. This allows nurses to monitor the progress of the wound while identifying the dominant tissue type.

A pale or grey-coloured wound bed can indicate unhealthy tissue. This is usually associated with chronic wounds with delayed healing.

Exudate

Wound exudate is the fluid that is produced by wounds. Noting the *type* and *amount* of exudate assists nurses to determine wound status.

Type of exudate

Normal exudate is pale-yellow in colour. Contaminants (such as bacteria) can result in discolouration. Exudates can be described as (Carville 2001):

- *serous*—clear fluid, straw-coloured fluid;
- *haemoserous*—slightly blood-stained serous fluid;
- *sanguineous*—heavily blood-stained fluid (or frank blood); or
- *purulent*—pus-containing fluid.

A combination of these terms can be used—for example, 'serosanguineous'.

Amount of exudate

Although serous fluid has a vital role in wound healing, the ideal wound surface is 'moist', rather than 'dry' or 'wet' (Thomas 1997).

The quantity of exudate determines the choice of dressing. However, it is difficult to be precise in documenting the amount of exudate—which is usually described as 'low', 'moderate', or 'heavy'. Because there is no simple, reliable, and accurate method of quantifying such terms, it must be acknowledged that there will be some variation among assessors.

Odour

Although most wounds have a smell associated with them, an offensive odour usually indicates the presence of high levels of bacteria. The presence of a putrid smell in combination with necrotic tissue indicates infection with anaerobic bacteria (Morison et al. 1997).

If possible, bacteria should be specifically identified by microscopy and culture. The infection should then be treated appropriately with systemic antibiotics, topical antimicrobials, and/or wound debridement.

Odour-reducing dressings (such as those containing charcoal) can be useful for certain types of wounds—for example, fungating wounds.

However, rather than masking the odour with a dressing, it is preferable to identify and eliminate the *cause* of the odour.

Surrounding skin

The skin surrounding a wound can develop a number of problems. If these are not detected and treated early, skin breakdown can occur. It is important to assess (and document) the problems presented in Table 3.3 (below).

Table 3.3 Problems of surrounding skin
AUTHOR'S PRESENTATION (ADAPTED FROM MORISON ET AL. 1997; MAKLEBUST & SIEGGREEN 2001; TENNANT 2000)

Problem	Description	Comments
Maceration	Soft, white, moist skin	Caused by exposure to excess moisture
Erythema	Redness (might or might not blanch when pressed)	Erythema can indicate infection or pressure Non-blanchable erythema is an early sign of tissue destruction
Contact dermatitis	Rash; dry, scaly, itchy skin	Can result from sensitivity to a dressing product, prolonged use of adhesive dressings or tapes, or prolonged exposure of the skin to wound exudate Management involves correct identification and elimination of the cause
Callus	Localised overgrowth of the horny layer of the epidermis	Usually an early indicator of pressure Occurs most commonly on the foot Cause of the pressure should be identified and eliminated Callus can mask a wound Removal of callus by experienced health professional is recommended
Induration	Hardness around a wound	Can be the result of tissue damage from radiotherapy or due to fibrosis associated with a chronic wound

Skin eruptions

If a nurse is to describe skin eruptions accurately, he or she requires a clear understanding of the terminology used to describe these conditions. The Box on page 47 provides a list of some commonly used terms and their definitions.

Terminology in skin eruptions

- *macule:* flat discolouration (brown, blue, red, or whitish) with a defined margin
- *plaque:* elevated, superficial, solid lesion with a defined margin greater than 0.5 cm in diameter; can be formed by a collection of papules
- *pustule:* collection of leucocytes and fluid with a defined margin; size can vary
- *papule:* elevated, solid lesion up to 0.5 cm in diameter
- *nodule:* elevated, solid lesion greater than 0.5 cm in diameter; the term 'tumour' might be used to describe a large nodule
- *vesicle:* collection of fluid with a defined margin up to 0.5 cm diameter
- *wheal:* firm, oedematous plaque caused by fluid infiltrating the dermis; can be short-lived; often due to an allergy

ADAPTED FROM BENBOW (2002)

Skin eruptions can be a manifestation of a disease process or health condition (for example, an allergy). The cause of skin eruptions should be investigated, and appropriate treatment instigated.

Linking assessment to practice

Long-term objectives

Comprehensive assessment of the person with a wound assists nurses to identify the long-term wound-management objective. This determines the appropriate choice of dressings and other interventions to promote wound healing.

Depending on the aetiology of the wound, management oriented towards the achievement of long-term objectives includes consideration of:

- choosing appropriate dressings;
- improving nutrition;
- reducing weight;
- relieving pressure;

- lifestyle changes (for example, cessation of smoking);
- control of other health conditions (for example, diabetes);
- review of medication;
- control of pain;
- new footwear;
- wearing of compression bandages; and
- referral to other healthcare professionals.

Short-term objectives

Through assessment of the wound itself, nurses identify short-term objectives. The wound assessment identifies which dressings are appropriate for the wound characteristics.

Regular, planned, systematic, documented re-assessment of the wound informs nurses of the wound's response to the management regimen. In general, if a particular wound-management regimen has been in place for four weeks without meeting the short-term objectives, a reassessment should be undertaken.

'If a particular regimen has been in place for four weeks without meeting the short-term objectives, a reassessment should be undertaken.'

If a change in the dressing regimen alone does not result in wound improvement, further investigation is required to rule out any previously undetected factors that might impair healing. The case study in the Box on page 49 provides an example of the need for a comprehensive reassessment if a wound does not progress as expected towards the achievement of short-term goals.

Introduction of a wound-assessment chart

Careful planning is required if a wound-assessment chart is to be introduced. This involves organisational support and the provision of education to assist nurses to accept the introduction of such a chart.

There are numerous types of charts available. Charts that are consistent with other forms of organisational documentation are the most effective (Massie 1998).

> ## Undetected diabetes
>
> A 60-year-old woman was admitted to hospital with an infected left hand following a scratch from a rose thorn.
>
> She was commenced on intravenous antibiotics and the wound was surgically debrided. Despite the antibiotics and frequent dressings the wound did not improve.
>
> Further investigations were therefore undertaken. It was discovered that the woman had diabetes mellitus—of which she was previously unaware.
>
> Once she was commenced on oral hypoglycaemic agents and an appropriate diet, her wound improved rapidly.

The process of introducing any new tool begins with a recognition that it is necessary. Once ideas have been developed regarding the information required in the chart, draft charts should be developed. To encourage acceptance, it is important to involve the nurses who will be the users of the final chart.

Following feedback on the use of the initial charts, a final draft chart should be designed. A trial period is then undertaken during which nurses have the opportunity to use the chart and provide further feedback. Once feedback is received and analysed, the tool is adjusted if necessary.

Finally, an implementation plan should be developed. Implementation might include structured education, changes to policies or guidelines, informal education, and modelling (Massie 1998).

Conclusion

Assessment is a vital component of wound management. It requires knowledge of the wound-healing process and the factors that can promote and impair wound healing.

A comprehensive assessment considers individual health, social and psychological status, and the characteristics of the wound itself.

This provides a sound foundation upon which wound-management interventions can be planned and implemented to achieve optimal outcomes for the person with a wound.

Acknowledgment

Parts of this chapter are adapted from an original article by the present author (Templeton 2003). The author gratefully acknowledges that permission to adapt and reproduce parts of the original article has been granted by the copyright holder, Royal District Nursing Service SA Inc. <www.rdns.net.au>.

Chapter 4
Dressings
Sue Templeton

Introduction

Just as every person is different, every wound is different. Each wound-management regimen must therefore be individually tailored in conjunction with the patient to meet his or her needs.

In modern wound management, dressings facilitate an optimal local wound environment to promote healing. However, dressings form only one component of an overall wound-management regimen. A comprehensive plan that is firmly based on the principles of modern wound management is more likely to have positive outcomes than one that focuses only on the dressings used.

The principles of wound management are:

- identify wound aetiology (cause);
- identify and (if possible) control or eliminate factors that can impair healing;
- set long-term and short-term objectives;
- implement a management regimen;

- review and revise the management regimen regularly and frequently; and
- achieve optimal outcomes.

(See Chapter 2, 'The Skin and Healing', page 15, for more on the principles of wound management, and Chapter 3, 'Assessment and Documentation', page 33, for a comprehensive discussion of assessment.)

In many instances the dressing is 'blamed' if a wound does not heal. However, many wounds fail to heal because the aetiology of the wound has not been identified or because factors that impair healing have not been controlled. In addition, for some patients, healing is not a realistic outcome. Rather than expect dressings to achieve rapid healing in every instance, dressings should be chosen with a view to achieving realistic objectives in view of the aetiology of the wound and its particular characteristics.

'Rather than expect dressings to achieve rapid healing in every instance, dressings should be chosen with a view to achieving realistic objectives.'

This chapter discusses the role and function of wound dressings. The chapter presumes that the other necessary components of wound management have been identified—and addressed in an appropriate manner.

Moist wound healing

George Winter is credited with laying the foundations of moist wound healing. Winter (1962) demonstrated a statistically significant difference in the rate of epithelialisation of standardised wounds in pigs. In Winter's study, wounds that had been covered with a polythene film epithelialised more rapidly than those that had been exposed to air. Since Winter's study, many similar studies have provided conclusive evidence that maintaining a moist wound environment achieves faster epithelialisation than does a dry wound environment (Parnham 2002).

'... conclusive evidence that maintaining a moist wound environment achieves faster epithelialisation than does a dry wound environment.'

The benefits of a moist wound environment include (ConvaTec 1999):

- reduced infection rates;
- reduced incidence of trauma and re-injury to the wound bed;
- enhanced autolytic debridement (selective to devitalised tissue);
- maintenance of growth factors at the wound surface; and
- enhanced stimulation of cell proliferation, collagen synthesis, and blood-vessel growth.

The 'ideal' wound dressing

Objectives

To facilitate an optimal local healing environment, an 'ideal' wound dressing (MacLellan & Rice 1995, Sibbald et al. 2000):

- controls exudate to achieve and maintain a moist wound environment;
- prevents maceration of the peri-wound skin;
- eliminates any dead space (by loosely filling cavities and sinuses);
- maintains optimal wound temperature;
- maintains optimal wound pH;
- prevents contamination with microorganisms;
- allows gaseous exchange;
- is free from particulate matter or toxic components; and
- is acceptable to the patient.

Moist wound environment

Dressings that regulate wound moisture are recommended. In choosing an appropriate dressing product, it is therefore imperative to ascertain the amount of wound exudate accurately. An effective dressing should prevent either maceration or desiccation.

Maceration is excessive moisture in the peri-wound skin. It can lead to excoriation and further wound breakdown (Collins, Hampton & White 2002).

Desiccation is drying-out of the wound. Desiccation can result in delayed healing and damage to underlying structures (such as tendon and bone).

Wound temperature

Dressings should provide thermal insulation to keep wound temperature at 37 degrees Celsius. A slight reduction in wound temperature (even as little as one degree Celsius) can delay healing (AWMA 2002).

To maintain a wound temperature close to body temperature, nurses should avoid prolonged exposure of the wound without a dressing. Application of cold solutions should also be avoided. During medical rounds to review wound progress, dressings should be left off for the shortest possible time.

Barrier to infection

An effective dressing provides a barrier to colonisation by bacteria. Occlusive dressings have a moisture-repellent backing—usually in the form of a film coating. This allows patients to shower, and is an effective barrier to bacterial penetration.

Some clinicians avoid using occlusive dressings because they believe that such dressings provide an ideal environment for multiplication of anaerobic microorganisms. However, these concerns have been refuted by experimental and clinical research (Jones & Milton 2000a).

Comfort and patient education

'Unresolved pain negatively affects wound healing and has an impact on quality of life' (WUWHS 2004). A moist wound environment is more comfortable for the patient because exposed nerve endings that are kept moist produce less discomfort and pain (Carville 2001).

Other factors that can affect comfort include:

- patient characteristics, preferences, and lifestyle;
- factors related to wound aetiology; and
- the dressing regimen.

Dressings should be chosen in conjunction with patients. Involving patients as partners in their care promotes acceptance of the suggested treatment and increases patient adherence with the regimen.

The patient's degree of comfort while wearing the dressing is affected by the number of layers used in the dressing, the composition of the dressing, and the techniques used in applying the dressing. There are still some patients and health professionals who believe that simple dry dressings are adequate for wound healing. These persons require education regarding the advantages of moist wound healing.

> *'Involving patients as partners in their care promotes acceptance of the suggested treatment and increases patient adherence with the regimen.'*

Dressings should not adhere to the wound bed because this can cause discomfort, delay healing, and traumatise the wound bed on removal (MacLellan & Rice 1995). The most common reason for dressing adhesion is inappropriate choice of dressing.

Leakage of exudate from dressings should also be avoided if possible. This can cause distress and soiling of clothing and bed linen. It also provides a potential portal of entry for microorganisms.

Choosing a dressing

Functionality of dressing products

There is a vast array of dressings available, and new dressings are always being developed and released. When choosing a dressing product, nurses should be aware of the following:

- the *purpose* of the dressing;
- the *specific characteristics* of the dressing—including how the dressing will behave when it is applied and how it handles exudate;
- the *correct application* of the dressing—including the amount of overlap onto peri-wound skin, whether a secondary dressing is required, and whether a particular side should be placed against the wound;

- whether a *secondary dressing* is required—for some occlusive dressings the application of a film over the entire dressing affects dressing performance; and

- the *expected wear time* of the dressing—this varies according to the amount of exudate, but there is usually a recommended time that is appropriate for each dressing.

Before using a particular dressing, nurses should familiarise themselves with the manufacturer's recommendations regarding the use and application of the dressing.

Exudate

To achieve moist wound healing, dressings should be chosen to regulate the amount of moisture at the wound. For example, a *dry* type of dressing (such as a calcium alginate) should be applied to *wet* (or high-exudate) wounds, whereas a *moist* type of dressing (such as a hydrogel) should be applied to *dry* (or low-exudate wounds). Figure 4.1 (below) provides an overview of choosing a dressing according to the amount of exudate.

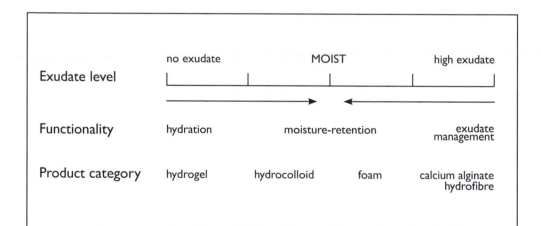

Figure 4.1 Choosing dressings to produce a moist environment
AUTHOR'S PRESENTATION (ADAPTED AND REPRODUCED FROM CARMODY & FORSTER 2003; PUBLISHED WITH PERMISSION)

Changing a choice of dressing

In most instances, no single dressing will be suitable for the life of the wound. Nurses should choose a dressing that is suitable for the patient and the wound at a particular time. In general, a dressing product should be used for about four weeks.

In choosing and using a dressing, nurses should ensure that:

- the choice is based on sound, evidence-based practice;
- the choice is consistent with the long-term wound-management objective;
- the wound characteristics have not changed (for example, level of exudate increasing or decreasing);
- the patient has not developed a sensitivity to the product;
- the wound has not become infected; and
- the dressing continues to suit the patient's requirements and the care setting.

If it is necessary to change the choice of dressing, the reasons for changing the dressing regimen should be carefully documented.

Cost-effectiveness of dressings

Moist wound-healing products are more expensive than traditional products (such as paraffin-impregnated gauze and ribbon gauze). However, when considering the cost of dressings, other factors should also be considered. The cost of nursing time involved in changing dressings, and other indirect costs (such as increased hospitalisation), are often overlooked (Bolton, Van Rijswijk & Shaffer 1996). For example, a saline-soaked dressing can require changing up to four times a day. In contrast, a moist wound-healing dressing (such as a hydrocolloid) can be left in place for up to seven days. A reduction in the frequency of dressing changes reduces the cost of nursing time, minimises interruption to the moist wound environment, minimises wound cooling, and frees up nursing time (that can be utilised in other activities).

In choosing a cost-effective dressing regimen the long-term objectives must be considered. In some circumstances, the use of a relatively costly dressing regimen for a short time can provide local conditions that accelerate healing significantly. Examples of this include the use of negative-pressure therapy or antimicrobial dressings. (For more information on negative-pressure therapy, see Chapter 9, 'Reconstructive Techniques', page 133; for more on antimicrobial dressings, see 'Antimicrobial dressings', this chapter, page 64.)

In dealing with a wound in which healing is *not* the objective, an inexpensive, comfortable, and easy dressing regimen that is acceptable to the patient and nurses might be appropriate.

Types of dressings

The following discussion focuses on the most commonly used types of products and on some products useful for specific clinical situations. The text discusses the types of dressings listed in the Box below.

Types of dressings
The text discusses the following types of dressings:
- dressings for hydration—hydrogels (page 58);
- dressings for moisture retention (page 60);
- dressings for exudate management (page 62);
- antimicrobial dressings (page 64);
- absorbent dressings (page 67); and
- inert dressings (page 68).

1. Dressings for hydration—hydrogels

Dry wounds (with low amounts of exudate) require a dressing that *adds* moisture to the wound bed. The most effective hydrating products are *hydrogels*. These dressings have a high water content in insoluble polymers (Sibbald et al. 2000).

In dry or low-exudate wounds, hydrogels promote debridement through autolysis. Hydrogels are contraindicated in wounds with moderate-to-high exudate because they can cause maceration. Hydrogels should not be used in sinuses (Carville 2001).

Hydrogels are available in various presentations, as listed in the Box below. These are discussed in the text that follows.

Dressings for hydration

The text discusses the following types of dressings for hydration:

- amorphous hydrogels;
- sheets of hydrogel;
- impregnated hydrogel dressings;
- hypertonic hydrogels.

Amorphous hydrogels

Amorphous hydrogels usually come in a tube. They can be spread onto the wound or used to fill a cavity, and require a secondary dressing to prevent the hydrogel drying out. Suitable secondary dressings include foam, paraffin-impregnated gauze, or hydrocolloid. A covering dressing might also be required—for example, a non-adherent dressing or combine.

The composition and consistency of hydrogels varies among brands. Most do not contain a preservative. However, some contain a preservative and are registered for multiple uses.

Sheets of hydrogel

Sheets of hydrogel are usually transparent sheets of hydrogel with the consistency of firm jelly. They are covered on one side with a film, and are available with or without an adhesive border.

Sheets of hydrogel can be useful for areas in which an amorphous hydrogel might become dry or 'squish' out (for example, under a bandage or on a surface such as the back of the leg).

Impregnated hydrogel dressings

These dressings have hydrogel impregnated into a carrier—usually non-woven gauze. They are useful for cavity wounds in which it is difficult to maintain the integrity of an amorphous hydrogel.

Hypertonic hydrogels

A hypertonic hydrogel is useful for rapid removal of hard, dry necrotic tissue. Once the necrotic tissue has autolysed and been removed, this product should be ceased.

2. Dressings for moisture retention

Wounds with low-to-moderate exudate require a dressing that will not dry out. However, the dressing should have some absorptive capacity. There are several dressing types in this category. These are listed in the Box on page 61, and discussed in the text below.

Films

Film dressings are comprised of a semi-permeable elastic sheet of polyurethane, coated with a hypoallergenic acrylic adhesive on one side (Jones & Milton 2000a). The dressing adheres to the peri-wound skin, but not to the wound surface.

Film dressings vary in their moisture-vapour transfer rate (MVTR). This is the rate at which the dressing allows water to evaporate. Film dressings are primarily used for superficial wounds with little exudate, for protection of surgical sites, and for fixing other dressings. They are not suitable for wounds with moderate or heavy exudate because excessive exudate accumulates under the film and causes maceration (Jones & Milton 2000a).

To achieve adhesion, the peri-wound skin must be clean, dry, and relatively free of hair. Because films can cause pain and tear fragile skin, nurses should use caution and follow the manufacturer's recommendations when removing these dressings.

Hydrocolloids

Hydrocolloids are composed of carboxymethylcellulose, other polysaccharides, and proteins (Sibbald et al. 2000). Some hydrocolloids also contain calcium alginate to increase their absorptive capacity and wear time.

Hydrocolloids have some absorptive capacity. They can remain in place for up to seven days.

Dressings for moisture retention

The text discusses the following types of dressings for moisture retention:

- films;
- hydrocolloids;
- hydroselective dressings; and
- continuous-irrigation dressings.

Hydrocolloids are not appropriate for wounds with high exudate because maceration and/or dressing leakage can occur. They can promote autolysis of devitalised tissue. To achieve adhesion, the peri-wound skin must be clean, dry, and relatively free of hair.

Hydrocolloids are available as:

- sheets;
- paste; and
- powder.

Sheets

Sheets are flat, self-adhesive dressings. The surface of the dressing must be in contact with the wound bed. Adhesion is increased by warming the dressing before application. The dressing should overlap the wound onto the peri-wound skin by a margin of at least 2 centimetres.

On contact with wound exudate, hydrocolloids form a gel. The normal appearance of the dressing in-use should not be confused with purulent exudate (Carville 2001). Some dressings have features (such as colour change or lines printed on the dressing) that indicate when to change the dressing.

Paste

Paste is available in a tube. It is useful for filling small cavities in which exudate is light to moderate. A hydrocolloid sheet can be used over paste.

Hydrocolloid *wound* paste should not be confused with paste used in stomal therapy.

Powder

Because this is a dry product, hydrocolloid powder absorbs more exudate. It turns from a powder to a gel in the presence of exudate.

Hydrocolloid powder can be sprinkled on wounds and is a useful for treating minor bleeding and odour in malignant wounds (Carville 2001).

Hydroselective dressings

Hydroselective dressings usually come in sheets. They are comprised of polyurethane gel matrix and a polyurethane covering film. Unlike hydrocolloids, they do not break down into a gel.

Hydroselective dressings absorb moderate amounts of fluid, but leave a concentration of proteins at the wound bed (Achterberg, Welling & Meyer-Ingold 1996). This can lead to improved wound-healing outcomes.

Continuous-irrigation dressings

These specialised dressings consist of an absorbent pad with irrigating properties. The dressing is activated with an electrolyte solution. It irrigates, cleanses, and debrides the wound bed while absorbing exudate. Continuous-irrigation dressings require changing every 24 hours.

3. Dressings for exudate management

Wounds with moderate-to-high amounts of exudate require absorbent dressings. There are several dressing types within this category. They vary according to absorptive capacity, presentation, composition, and indications for use. They include the dressings listed in the Box on page 63, and discussed in the text below.

'Wounds with moderate-to-high amounts of exudate require absorbent dressings.'

Foams

Foam dressings are composed of polyurethane or silicone (Jones & Milton 2000b). Depending on their composition, they can absorb low to high amounts of exudate. They can be used as a primary or secondary dressing.

Foams are available as sheets and fillers.

Dressings for exudate management

The text discusses the following types of dressings for exudate management:

- foams;
- calcium alginates; and
- hydrofibres.

Sheets come in adhesive and non-adhesive forms. They vary according to the number of layers in the dressing and the amount of exudate they can absorb. Some foams have additional additives that exhibit distinctive properties.

Fillers are available in several presentations—including preformed cavity dressings, sheets, and two-part polymers. The polymers are mixed together, and then set to the wound shape.

Foam dressings provide good thermal insulation (Jones & Milton 2000b). They can provide extra padding or cushioning. However, they should not be used in place of appropriate pressure-reducing devices. Some have the ability to 'lock' fluid into the dressing matrix—making them useful under compression therapy.

Foam dressings are not suitable as a primary dressing for dry wounds. Silicone-coated foam dressings prevent adhesion at the wound surface, minimise pain during dressing changes, and minimise damage to wound tissue (Thomas 2003).

Calcium alginates

Calcium alginates are dressings primarily derived from brown kelp (seaweed) (Sibbald et al. 2000), and contain a polymer composed of varying amounts of guluronic and mannuronic acid (Pudner 1997).

When exudate comes into contact with a calcium alginate, the dressing becomes a gel. Some calcium alginates can assist in achieving haemostasis.

Calcium alginates are available as sheets and ropes.

Sheets are available in various thicknesses and presentations. Some types lose their form when wet; they then form a soft gel. Others have a tighter weave or are needle-bonded. This form retains its shape and structure, and forms a firm gel. Because the dressing is easily removed as one piece, firm-gelling calcium alginates are useful for filling sinuses and deep cavities.

Ropes are also available in various thicknesses and presentations.

Calcium alginates usually require a secondary dressing. They are not suitable for dry or low-exudate wounds because the dressing must form a gel to achieve a moist wound environment. In-use, the dressing should not be confused with purulent exudate or wound crust. Nurses should ensure that all dressing residue is removed by gently irrigating with saline.

Hydrofibres

Hydrofibre dressings have a similar appearance to calcium alginates. However, hydrofibre dressings are composed of sodium carboxymethylcellulose (Alderman 2004b). In contact with exudate, the dressing forms a firm gel.

Hydrofibre dressings are suitable for wounds with heavy exudate. The dressings absorb exudate only in a vertical pattern, and the peri-wound skin is therefore protected from maceration (Carville 2001).

Hydrofibre dressings are available in ropes and sheets and require a secondary dressing. They do not have haemostatic properties and are not suitable for dry or low-exudate wounds.

4. Antimicrobial dressings

Antimicrobial dressings are useful for wounds with high bacterial loads. They can be used in conjunction with systemic antibiotics to treat clinical infection.

Some antimicrobial dressings (such as cadexomer iodine or those that release silver) can be very effective as a component of wound-bed preparation. These dressings assist in overcoming high bacterial loads in wounds—which can contribute to diminished healing of certain chronic wounds. (Wound-bed preparation is discussed in detail in Chapter 6, 'Wound Bed Preparation', page 89.)

There are many antimicrobial dressings on the market, and nurses should investigate the particular properties of the dressing before choosing one. They are categorised according to their main antimicrobial component. These include the dressings listed in the Box below, and discussed in the text that follows.

Antimicrobial dressings

The text discusses the following types of antimicrobial dressings:

- topical antibiotics;
- povidone-iodine;
- cadexomer iodine;
- silver;
- hypertonic saline impregnated dressings; and
- medical honey.

Topical antibiotics

Topical antibiotics are available as creams, ointments, and impregnated sheets. Topical antibiotics are usually of limited clinical use in wound management. The exception to this is silversulphadiazine cream, which is still used in many settings—particularly to treat *Pseudomonas aeruginosa* (Lansdown 2002).

Povidone-iodine

Povidone-iodine is available as a solution, an ointment, and in impregnated sheets. Povidone-iodine dressings are used for treatment of low-exudate, infected wounds. The iodine is rapidly broken down, and dressing changes should therefore be carried out at least daily (Jones & Milton 2000c).

Anecdotal evidence suggests that persons with arterial insufficiency respond well to povidone-iodine. There is continuing debate as to whether povidone-iodine is appropriate for wound management.

Cadexomer iodine

This dressing incorporates cadexomer spheres containing 0.9% water-soluble iodine (Falanga 1997). Cadexomer iodine is different from povidone-iodine. As exudate is taken into a cadexomer-iodine dressing, it swells and forms a gel—thus releasing iodine (Falanga 1997). The dressing slowly releases iodine for up to three days. A secondary dressing is required.

Cadexomer iodine effectively debrides devitalised tissue. Because exudate is required to release the iodine, cadexomer iodine is suitable for moderate-to-high exudate wounds.

Cadexomer iodine is available as paste, sheets, and powder. There are some precautions of which nurses should be aware, and the manufacturer's information should be checked before using cadexomer iodine.

Silver

Silver is a fast-acting, broad-spectrum, effective antimicrobial (Wright, Lam & Burrell 1998), and there are many dressings that contain silver. Some of these release silver onto the wound, whereas others kill bacteria absorbed into the dressing.

'Silver is a fast-acting, broad-spectrum, effective antimicrobial.'

For wound management, the most effective silver is delivered in an ionic or nanocrystalline form (Lansdown 2002). Because topical silver treats only the wound surface (Sibbald et al. 2000), the efficacy of silver dressings can be reduced if dressings are applied over thick slough or necrotic tissue.

Sustained-release silver dressings are available in numerous forms, and nurses should choose one that suits the characteristics of the wound being treated.

Hypertonic saline-impregnated dressings

These dressings create an osmotic action that cleanses the wound by drawing in necrotic tissue and purulent debris (Carville 2001).

Hypertonic saline dressings are useful for moderate-to-high exudate wounds with slough and purulent exudate. They require dressing changes at least every day.

There are specific considerations regarding the use of these dressings, and the manufacturer's instructions should be followed.

Medical honey

Honey from certain *Leptospermum* species has been demonstrated to have antibacterial, anti-inflammatory, and debriding actions (Templeton 2001). The antibacterial effects of honey are attributed to its high osmolarity and the sustained release of low-dose hydrogen peroxide as the honey becomes diluted with exudate (Templeton 2001).

Honey requires dressing changes at least every day. Wounds with high exudate might require dressing changes three times per day (Carville 2001).

> '*Honey has been demonstrated to have antibacterial, anti-inflammatory, and debriding actions.*'

5. Absorbent dressings

Depending on their presentation and composition, absorbent dressings can be used as primary or secondary dressings. As secondary dressings they can be valuable for moderate-to-high exudate wounds if the primary dressing is not able to contain all the exudate. They can prevent leakage of exudate and reduce the frequency of dressing changes.

Absorbent dressings include multi-layer dressings and absorbent pads.

Multi-layer dressings can be used as primary or secondary dressings. They are available in adhesive and non-adhesive forms. Some have a film backing—making them waterproof. Some contain highly absorbent granules or beads that swell and 'lock' exudate into them.

> '*Absorbent dressings can be used as primary or secondary dressings.*'

Absorbent pads are usually used as secondary dressings. They contain a dense, highly absorbent pulp core that retains large amounts of exudate. Some have a water-repellent backing, and others have a non-shear wound-contact layer.

6. Inert dressings

Inert dressings do *not* interact with the wound bed to create a moist wound environment. Inert dressings include gauze, paraffin-impregnated tulle dressings, petrolatum-emulsion dressings, silicone sheets, and 'non-adherent' dressings.

Inert dressings are usually used for wounds that are healing by primary intention, for protection of newly healed skin or skin grafts, or as secondary dressings (Alderman 2004a). However, there are some circumstances in which inert dressings are appropriate as primary wound dressings.

'Inert dressings are usually used for wounds that are healing by primary intention, for protection of newly healed skin, or as secondary dressings.'

Some so-called 'non-adherent' dressings can become adherent to the wound bed—particularly if they are not changed frequently.

Conclusion

Dressings form one component of a comprehensive wound-management regimen. Nurses are well positioned to assess, choose, and evaluate dressings.

It is easy to become confused by the vast array of products that are available. In clinical practice, nurses can appropriately manage most wounds with a basic range of products. For many wounds, any one of several dressings might be appropriate. However, specialised products are necessary in certain circumstances.

'With knowledge, creativity, and innovation, nurses can optimise clinical outcomes for a person with a wound.'

Although there is much debate among clinicians about the usefulness and appropriateness of certain dressings, nurses are encouraged to 'never say never'. There are always clinical situations in which the choice of a dressing might seem to be unusual. However, each patient and each wound must be considered individually. With knowledge, creativity, and innovation, nurses can optimise clinical outcomes for a person with a wound.

Chapter 5

Cleansing and Skin Care

Therese Chand

Introduction

Effective wound management requires removal of debris and foreign bodies from wound tissue. Until the wound is clean, inflammation persists and optimum wound healing cannot occur.

The general term 'wound cleansing' can be taken to include everything from removal of foreign bodies, to debridement, to the use of antimicrobials. Although there have been many developments in the field of wound care, there remains a lack of consensus about 'wound cleansing'—including which cleansing agent is superior and which method is the most appropriate for the patient's needs.

'Until the wound is clean, inflammation persists and optimum wound healing cannot occur.'

When considering the treatment of a wound, it is important to ask certain questions. These include:

- Does the wound need cleansing?
- What will be gained by cleaning the wound?
- What method or technique would be most appropriate?

This chapter canvasses these issues according to the framework outlined in the Box below.

General principles of wound cleansing

Wound cleansing is the process of removing debris, bacteria, foreign material, and exudate from a wound surface. The goal is to create an environment that enhances wound healing by removing debris and contaminants from the wound bed without damaging healthy or newly formed tissue.

In cleansing wounds, nurses should remove only as much as is necessary to prevent infection. The aim is to remove foreign bodies, excess exudate, debris, slough, and necrotic tissue that might become a focus for infection. The infection-control guidelines of the healthcare facility should be consulted and followed.

'Wound cleansing is the process of removing debris, bacteria, foreign material, and exudate from a wound surface.'

The benefits of facilitating wound healing must be balanced against the damage that can result from cleansing. Damage to tissues is not always obvious; it often occurs at the cellular level without macroscopic manifestations. Nurses must be aware that toxicity from cleansing solutions can outweigh the potential benefit. It is therefore important to understand the properties of the solutions in assessing the type of solution to be used, the frequency of cleansing, and the method of cleansing (swabbing, irrigation, bathing).

A summary of the most important principles of wound healing is presented in the Box below.

> ## General principles of wound cleansing
> The most important general principles of wound cleansing can be summarised as follows:
> - determine the appropriate type of cleansing solution;
> - choose the most effective method of cleansing;
> - minimise chemical irritation;
> - minimise mechanical trauma; and
> - consider the individual needs of patients.

Aseptic technique and clean technique

When choosing the technique and method of cleansing, nurses must first make a thorough assessment of the patient's needs. The advantages and disadvantages of treatment regimens must be carefully weighed before treatment is implemented. Decisions must be based on current expert opinion and best evidence.

In general, wound-cleansing techniques can be categorised as:
- aseptic technique; or
- clean technique.

Aseptic ('sterile') technique is indicated for surgical wounds, traumatic wounds, and infected wounds. *Clean* technique is usually required for chronic wounds in healthy patients.

Aseptic technique

Asepsis is the prevention of microbial contamination by excluding, removing, or killing microorganisms. Aseptic technique (often called 'sterile' technique) is the use of practices aimed at preventing pathological organisms entering the body. When applied to wound management, aseptic technique is the prevention of pathological microorganisms entering the body through an open wound.

The procedures followed in surgical operations represent the best-known example of aseptic technique. These include:

- *equipment procedures:* absolute sterilisation of all instruments, surgical drapes, and other inanimate objects that might come into contact with the surgical wound; and
- *personnel procedures:* personnel (such as surgeons and nurses) washing their hands for at least five minutes with a germicidal soap and wearing sterile surgical gloves and gowns to avoid wound contamination.

When applied to wound care, aseptic technique implies the use of sterile equipment that might come into contact with the wound during wound cleansing. This equipment includes scissors, dressings, single-use solutions, gloves, and other inanimate objects.

Clean technique

Clean technique ensures that the wound, dressings, and all fields are free of dirt or obvious soiling. This involves measures that reduce the potential of introducing microorganisms—such as the avoidance of direct contact with the susceptible site.

'Clean technique involves measures that reduce the potential of introducing microorganisms—such as the avoidance of direct contact with the susceptible site.'

Clean technique follows sound infection-control principles to prevent transmission of pathogens. It utilises clean (rather than sterile) single-use gloves and tap water (safe for drinking). This technique is suitable for such wound-management procedures as irrigation of chronic wounds in a community setting.

Choosing aseptic or clean technique

There is a lack of consensus on the question of when to use aseptic technique and when to use clean technique. Several studies have reported that there is no evidence to suggest that sterile technique provides a better healing outcome (Stotts et al. 1997; Faller 1997). However, it has been suggested that 'the level of asepsis should increase as the procedure becomes more invasive' (Crow 1997, pp 93–4). It also appears that the knowledge and skill level of healthcare providers affect decisions regarding the level of asepsis required (Crow 1997).

The costs associated with dressing changes using clean technique are significantly less than those associated with changes using sterile technique. It is important to remember that most wounds are already colonised by microorganisms, and that the objective of wound cleansing and debridement is to reduce the amount of necrotic material and debris that supports bacterial growth and delays wound healing. This is particularly true with chronic wounds.

'Most wounds are already colonised by microorganisms.'

Variables such as age, general health, immune status, psychosocial status, and type of wound must all be taken into account in making a decision about the technique to be employed. In addition, a hospital setting is different from a home environment, and structured hospital guidelines for wound cleansing and dressing might not be applicable in a home situation. Each situation needs to be assessed individually. However, the *principles* of asepsis should be applied, regardless of the practice setting.

'The principles of asepsis should be applied, regardless of the practice setting.'

Wound-cleansing methods

Wound cleansing is performed to remove (or loosen) foreign materials from the wound bed. To achieve this, the volume of cleansing solution must be adequate and the solution must be delivered with adequate pressure.

Regardless of what type of solution is used, nurses must ensure that the solution is at body temperature. A low temperature can impede cellular mitotic activity and adversely affect the availability of oxygen in the wound (Young 1995).

A variety of wound-cleansing solutions is now available. If nurses are to select the most appropriate solution for a specific situation, they require an understanding of the characteristics and actions of these various products.

In carrying out cleansing, the following methods can be employed:
- swabbing and/or debridement;
- irrigation; and
- bathing.

This is illustrated in Figure 5.1, below. These methods are discussed in more detail in the text that follows.

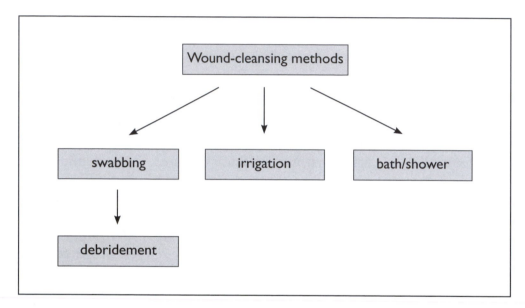

Figure 5.1 Wound-cleansing methods
Author's presentation

Wound swabbing and/or debridement

Wound swabbing is controversial because swabbing can redistribute the bacteria and drive them deeper into the tissues where they can act as a focus for infection (Thomlinson 1987; Ovington 2001; Blunt 2001).

Wound swabbing can also shed fibres from cotton wool or gauze. These can cause a prolonged inflammatory response and increased risk of infection.

Pressure caused by swabbing can damage newly formed or granulating tissue—again prolonging healing time.

For infected wounds, physical removal of thick materials might require wound debridement. This is discussed in more detail in Chapter 6, 'Wound Bed Preparation', page 89.

Irrigation

Irrigation, sometimes called 'lavage', is the preferred method for cleansing wounds—particularly traumatic wounds in which cleansing is likely to require large volumes of fluid to remove debris. In contrast to swabbing, this method means that there is no risk of fibres being shed into the wound.

The main purpose of irrigation is to remove bacteria—rather than kill them. Wound irrigation can also be used to: (i) remove foreign bodies and debris; (ii) remove excessive exudate, blood, and necrotic tissue; and (iii) provide moisture.

'Irrigation is the preferred method for cleansing wounds.'

The main concern with respect to irrigation is uncertainty regarding the amount of pressure that should be used. Inadequate pressure is ineffective in removing exudate and loose tissue (Oliver 1997; Williams 1999). In contrast, excessive pressure can cause damage to delicate granulation tissue. A pressure of 4–15 pounds per square inch (approx. 200–800 mm Hg) should be used to reduce the risk of trauma and wound infection (Bergstrom et al. 1994).

Irrigation can be performed using a syringe (without a needle), a rubber-bulb syringe, or pre-packed irrigation systems.

The common solutions used for irrigation are normal saline, tap water, or topical antiseptic solutions (for example, chlorhexidine and iodine).

Bathing

The third method of wound cleansing is bathing. Before using bathing to cleanse a wound, nurses should consider:

- the suitability of the wound for bathing;
- the type of skin closure used; and
- the patient's situation and preferences.

Each of these is discussed below.

Suitability of the wound

Chronic wounds and wounds that are likely to be already colonised with bacteria are suitable for bathing. This method of cleansing is often recommended for wounds that have been left to heal by secondary intention—such as pressure ulcers, perineal wounds, and pilonidal sinuses. It is becoming increasingly common for chronic wounds (such as leg ulcers) to be cleansed in a bath or shower.

'Chronic wounds and wounds that are likely to be already colonised with bacteria are suitable for bathing.'

In addition to cleansing the wound and the surrounding skin, bathing has the added benefit of allowing adherent dressings to be soaked off, thus increasing ease of removal. Bathing can also be of great psychological benefit to the patient (Morison 1998; Fernandez, Griffiths & Ussia 2002).

Type of skin closure

In the case of surgical wounds, the type of skin closure should be considered. A continuous subcuticular suture is unlikely to pose an increased risk of infection, but interrupted sutures (such as silk) provide a wick by which microorganisms can enter the wound.

Patient's situation and preferences

Careful consideration must be given to each patient's individual situation, needs, and preferences. Healing can be affected by age, medications, site of wound, and underlying disease. Persons with diabetes who have leg ulcers are advised not to bathe their wounds because of the increased risk of infection.

Physical problems in accessing bathing facilities, such as poor mobility, can be overcome by wheelchair-access bathrooms and equipment such as hoists, lifters, and shower chairs. Restrictions on bathing at home should be assessed, and appropriate equipment and aids can be obtained as required.

Certain cultural and religious beliefs might prohibit the bathing of wounds, and these should be respected.

If economic considerations are relevant, it should be remembered that readily available tap water is cheaper than manufactured supplies of saline. However, the use of tap water as cleansing solution is dependent on the water coming from a properly treated supply.

Antimicrobial agents

The two main groups of antimicrobial agents used in wound management are *antiseptics* and *antibiotics*. Each has specific characteristics in dealing with the bacterial load in a wound bed.

Antiseptics

General comments on antiseptics

Antiseptics are solutions that inhibit the growth of microorganisms. In contrast, a *germicide* is a chemical that kills bacteria outright. The term 'antiseptic' can also include disinfectants, but most disinfectants are too strong to be applied to body tissues and are therefore generally used to clean inanimate objects (such as trolleys, floors, and bathroom fixtures).

The use of antiseptics in wound care is based on the belief that they help to remove bacteria from the surface of open wounds—thus reducing exudate and odour, and encouraging healing. However, although antiseptics have been used to treat wounds for decades, their use is controversial because of concerns that they might be toxic to normal wound tissues (Leaper 1996). Granulation tissue and fibroblasts are most susceptible to cytotoxic damage by antiseptics. The benefits and risks of using any given antiseptic must therefore be carefully assessed, particularly if it is to be used frequently or for a prolonged period.

'Although antiseptics have been used to treat wounds for decades, their use is controversial because they might be toxic to normal wound tissues.'

Antiseptics have a broad range of antimicrobial activity against both Gram-positive and Gram-negative species, as well as many fungi and viruses. This makes them potentially valuable in controlling bacterial levels in non-healing chronic wounds, which often have multiple microbial colonisation.

The effectiveness of antiseptics is related to their dilution and the duration of exposure to tissues. They need enough contact time with the microorganisms to be effective. However, most antiseptics are not in contact with the wound long enough to be effective and, if left for a longer period, they might cause damage to tissues.

'Most antiseptics are not in contact with the wound long enough to be effective.'

Some antiseptics are deactivated in the presence of organic matter (such as exudate, blood, and pus). These are clearly unsuitable for use in wound care. In addition, some antiseptics can cause hypersensitivity reactions in certain patients. In particular, povidone-iodine and chlorhexidine can cause hypersensitivity reactions (Lawrence 1998; Burks 1998).

The Box below summarises the factors that should be taken into account in choosing an appropriate antiseptic.

Choosing an appropriate antiseptic

This portion of the text has discussed several factors that should be taken into account in choosing an appropriate antiseptic. Nurses should choose an antiseptic that:

- is non-toxic to tissues;
- is effective against a wide range of organisms;
- is effective over a wide range of dilutions;
- does not cause hypersensitivity reactions;
- works rapidly (to minimise tissue exposure);
- is not deactivated in the presence of blood, pus, or exudate; and
- is relatively cheap.

ADAPTED FROM MORISON (1992)

The antiseptics most commonly used in wound care include the following:

- povidone–iodine;
- hydrogen peroxide;

- aqueous chlorhexidine solutions;
- chlorhexidine gluconate and cetrimide ('Savlon');
- sodium hypochlorite; and
- mercury compounds.

Each of these is discussed below.

Povidone-iodine

Povidone-iodine is effective against many species of Gram-positive and Gram-negative bacteria (including *Proteus spp*), fungi, and viruses. It is widely used in pre-operative and post-operative skin treatment, and as an effective cleansing solution for contaminated wounds (including burns). It is also used to cleanse skin before insertion of external tubes and ports. Slow-release iodine solution (cadexomer iodine) is effective for wounds colonised with MRSA.

'Iodine toxicity can occur ... povidone-iodine is not recommended for long-term wound cleansing.'

Povidone-iodine is available in a variety of commercial formulations—including lotions, creams, ointments, impregnated dressing products, and surgical soaps.

There are several disadvantages. Povidone-iodine is deactivated in the presence of organic materials (such as pus, blood, and exudate), and it is cytotoxic to fibroblasts in stronger concentrations. Its effects wear off after a relatively short time, and it does discolour the skin.

Absorption of iodine (and iodine toxicity) can occur in young children, in people with thyroid problems, and in people with poor renal function (Lineweaver 1985). Povidone-iodine is not recommended for long-term wound cleansing. If being used to wash wounds, povidone-iodine should be rinsed off after 3–5 minutes. Because of the potential for systemic absorption, it should not be used as packing in large wounds.

In addition, povidone-iodine can cause skin hypersensitivities; patients with skin sensitivity should be patch-tested before use (Karukonda et al. 2000).

Antiseptics

This portion of the text discusses selected antiseptics. The antiseptics discussed are:

- povidone–iodine (page 79);
- hydrogen peroxide (page 80);
- aqueous chlorhexidine solutions (page 81);
- chlorhexidine gluconate and cetrimide ('Savlon') (page 81);
- sodium hypochlorite (page 81); and
- mercury compounds (page 81).

Hydrogen peroxide

The effervescent cleansing action of hydrogen peroxide helps to lift debris from the wound surface. It converts to oxygen and water when it comes in contact with catalase—an enzyme found in blood and most tissues.

Hydrogen peroxide can deodorise infected wounds. It is useful in removing crusts around gastrostomy, nephrostomy, and tracheostomy sites. It is a relatively cheap antiseptic, and skin hypersensitivity is rare.

However, it is relatively weak, and is effective only in high concentrations. Such high concentrations can cause cytotoxic effects on fibroblasts and granulation tissue. Although higher concentrations are available, the appropriate concentration is a 3% solution.

'Hydrogen peroxide should not be used in wounds with sinus tracts or in closed cavities.'

Hydrogen peroxide should not be used in wounds with sinus tracts or in closed cavities where release of oxygen is impaired; this can cause air embolism. Hydrogen peroxide can dissolve clots—resulting in bleeding. Cotton 'buds' (or 'tips') should be used to apply hydrogen peroxide in the vicinity of pin sites and drain sites to ensure that the solution does not enter cavities.

After using hydrogen peroxide, nurses should rinse well with normal saline. Some patients can experience itchy sensations if not rinsed.

Aqueous chlorhexidine solution

Aqueous chlorhexidine is effective against a wide range of Gram-positive and Gram-negative bacteria. Its antibacterial activity against *Staphylococcus aureus* and *Pseudomonas aeruginosa* is important in clinical practice (Cooper 2004). It is not effective against acid-fast bacilli, bacterial spores, viruses, and fungi.

Although it has low toxicity, hypersensitivity reactions can occur. Aqueous chlorhexidine is inactivated by organic materials—such as pus, slough, and blood. It is also inactivated if used in conjunction with povidone-iodine solution.

Chlorhexidine gluconate and cetrimide ('Savlon')

These solutions are effective against Gram-positive and Gram-negative bacteria. They have emulsifying and detergent properties, and are effective in cleaning debris from contaminated wounds, particularly traumatic wounds.

Cetrimide is a preservative that is included in the product to extend product shelf-life. However, cetrimide can be toxic to fibroblasts and can cause skin irritation.

Contamination with *Pseudomonas aeruginosa* has been reported (Pirnay et al. 2000).

Sodium hypochlorite solutions ('Eusol', 'Milton', 'Dakin's solution')

The traditional use of hypochlorite solutions has been to remove slough by gauze packing of cavity wounds. However, hypochlorite solutions are cytotoxic to fibroblasts and impair epithelial migration. They are also much more alkaline than normal skin. Hypochlorite solutions have a working pH of 7.5–8.5, whereas skin pH is normally 4.5–5.5. Hypochlorite solutions are rapidly inactivated in the presence of organic fluids, unless used in high concentrations.

Mercury compounds

Mercury-based compounds are bacteriostatic and fungistatic—but only in high concentrations. They are not recommended for use in wounds, especially in children, because they can cause mercury toxicity, anaphylaxis, agranulocytosis, and aplastic anaemia (Dealey 1994).

Tap water and normal saline

Although tap water and normal saline are not antiseptics, it has been reported that no difference in infection rates and healing rates occurs in wounds that are cleansed with tap water or normal saline, rather than with antiseptics (Cochrane Library 2002).

Tap water

Cold tap water is recommended as first-aid management for cooling wounds immediately after burns. It is also used for cleansing traumatic wounds of debris. It is not usually recommended for patients with diabetes—due to risks of infection.

Showering with tap water is recommended for cleaning drain sites—especially in community settings. Nurses should run the water from the tap for several minutes before use to clear any standing water from the system.

Normal saline

Normal saline is the solution of choice for irrigation of wounds in hospital settings. Patients should be warned that it can cause slight discomfort when used in open wounds.

Antibiotics

Antibiotics are potent antimicrobial agents that either kill microorganisms or inhibit the reproduction of microorganisms.

Most wounds, especially chronic wounds, are colonised by microbes. All wounds have surface contamination—that is, the presence of bacteria without proliferation. In certain circumstances, these microorganisms can proliferate and invade tissues—thus producing an infection. It is important to differentiate between contamination and infection (see Chapter 6, page 89, for more on this). The clinical signs and symptoms of infection include inflammation, swelling, pus, fever, pain, change in exudate colour, and unusual odour.

If a wound is infected, it is important to treat it aggressively and appropriately. Management usually consists of a combined approach using appropriate systemic antibiotics and topical application of antibacterial agents (such as application of a suitable dressing with antibacterial activity).

Topical antibiotics are not recommended in all wound infections. They can cause hypersensitivity reactions or lead to the emergence of antibiotic-resistant strains of bacteria. However, in some cases they can be useful. The Box below summarises some of the more commonly used topical antibiotics.

In general, the routine use of antibiotics is discouraged. Treatment with antibiotics should be reserved for definite infections—as diagnosed clinically or by laboratory tests.

Topical antibiotics

Commonly prescribed topical antimicrobials include:

- gentamicin sulphate (effective against Gram-negative organisms)
- polymyxin B (effective against Gram-negative organisms)
- silver sulphadiazine (effective against Gram-positive and Gram-negative bacteria and *Candida*)
- neomycin (effective against Gram-positive organisms)
- mupirocin (effective against Gram-positive organisms, including MRSA)
- bacitracin (effective against Gram-positive organisms)

General skin care

A regular skin-care program, combined with a healthy diet, helps to keep skin supple and moist. A good skin-care program aims to:

- maintain the skin's normal pH;
- maintain skin hydration; and
- prevent skin breakdown.

This is especially important in the very young and the aged—in whom the protective properties of the skin are more likely to be compromised.

Products applied to the skin during skin cleansing must not contain chemicals that irritate the skin or damage its protective barrier. It is important that nurses be aware of the ingredients in each skin-care product. With this information, nurses are then well placed to choose a suitable product for:

- skin cleansing;
- moisturising; and
- protection.

Each of these is discussed below.

Skin-cleansing agents

Skin cleansers should provide fast, effective cleansing. There are now several cleansing products available that have a physiological pH (5.5). This helps to maintain the skin's natural defence barrier. Such cleansers, which contain surfactants to lift dirt and debris, are superior to soaps—because soap has an alkaline pH (7.0–11.0) that emulsifies the lipid coating of the skin. In addition, soap has other disadvantages—including the presence of perfumes and other caustic chemicals (which can irritate the skin) and other inorganic substances (which can leave a residue after washing).

Although new commercial soaps have added ingredients (such as coconut oil and glycerin) to 'replace' the skin's protective coating, the majority of soaps are still alkaline. Frequent and prolonged exposure to soap will thus compromise the skin's ability to maintain its normal acidity.

Moisturisers

A moisturiser is an agent that softens and soothes the skin by maintaining moisture levels. Moisturisers are usually made from a combination of water, lipids, and wax. They are essential products in managing dry and flaky skin.

General skin care

This portion of the text discusses general skin care. The subjects discussed are:

- skin cleansing;
- moisturising; and
- protection.

Moisturisers form a lipid film over the skin. This reduces water loss and increases moisture levels in the skin. This then restores the skin's elasticity and reduces pruritus caused by dryness.

For skin that is very dry or scaly, a moisturiser that is oil-based or emollient-based is more effective than a cream or lotion. Nurses should avoid using moisturisers with lanolin and perfumes—because these often cause hypersensitivity reactions.

Protection

Excessive moisture—due to perspiration, wound exudate, or incontinence—can put patients at risk of skin breakdown and the development of pressure ulcers. A build-up of moisture makes the skin more liable to water-soluble skin irritants, and can macerate the skin.

Incontinence is a particular risk. Prolonged exposure of the skin to urine can damage the skin because ammonia in the urine increases the pH of the skin to alkaline levels, and because organic salts and crystallised urine can irritate the skin. Exposure to faeces can macerate the skin and increase the bacterial load. To minimise the harmful effects of incontinence, the skin must be cleansed after each episode. Appropriate barrier creams on the perineum prevent direct and prolonged contact between the skin and the offending urine or faecal output.

'To minimise the harmful effects of incontinence, the skin must be cleansed after each episode.'

Excessive wound discharge must be contained using highly absorbent dressings or bagging. For patients who perspire freely, frequent changes of clothes and drying of skin might be necessary. Leakage from stomas (such as ileostomies and colostomies) must be attended to immediately, and appliances should be changed if required.

Care of denuded skin

Apart from the effects of maceration (as described above), other causes of denuded skin include:

- exposure to irritants (including skin-care products) causing hypersensitivity and contact dermatitis; and
- adhesive dressings, tapes, and electrodes—which can lift the top layer of skin when removed from patients with fragile skin (especially babies and the elderly).

The first step in treatment is to eliminate the offending product or adhesive—particularly those that require frequent stripping and removal.

There are several products that are specifically designed for treatment of denuded skin. Products containing karaya are useful because they adhere to skin and protect it—without aggravating the problem. Barrier wipes that leave a protective film on the skin can also be useful in some situations.

Conclusion

Bacteria can colonise (and potentially infect) any wound. To facilitate healing and improve a patient's overall condition, nurses must therefore take steps to control or reduce the number of bacteria present in a wound.

Key strategies to achieve this include:
- application of the principles of asepsis;
- the use of wound-cleansing agents;
- the use of antimicrobials (such as antiseptics and antibiotics); and
- the use of other appropriate skin-care products that can improve specific skin conditions.

To facilitate improved symptom control and better outcomes, it is the responsibility of every nurse to have a sound knowledge of the principles of asepsis and the properties of the available cleansing agents and other skin-care products.

Chapter 6

Wound Bed Preparation

Terry Swanson

Introduction

Wound-bed preparation (WBP) is increasingly recognised as being crucial to effective chronic wound management. Application of the proactive principles of WBP leads to the adoption of the best approach to the healing of chronic wounds and optimises the function of modern dressings and technologies.

> *'Wound-bed preparation is crucial to effective chronic wound management.'*

Definition and components of WBP

WBP can be defined as 'the promotion of wound closure through diagnosis of the cause, attention to patient-centered concerns, and correction of systemic and local factors that may delay healing' (Sibbald et al. 2003, p. 24).

The key components of WBP are (Sibbald et al. 2003; Chin, Shultz & Stacey 2003; Flanagan 2003):

- assessment of patient factors and wound factors;
- integration of the patient's needs and concerns into the management plan;

- implementation and monitoring of systemic and local treatment;
- management of non-viable tissue (debridement);
- management of inflammation and bacterial balance;
- management of wound exudate or moisture balance;
- correction of cellular dysfunction and restoration of biochemical balance;
- monitoring of wound edges and peri-wound areas for healing or complications;
- education of the patient; and
- collaboration of the healthcare team in providing evidence-based care.

Principles of WBP

The International Wound Bed Preparation Advisory Board has developed an acronym to facilitate knowledge and application of the principles of WBP (Schultz et al., 2003). The acronym is the word 'TIME', in which:

- *T* refers to 'tissue management' (debridement);
- *I* refers to 'infection' or 'inflammation';
- *M* refers to 'moisture imbalance'; and
- *E* refers to 'edge of wound'.

These four principles form the framework for most of the discussion of WBP that follows in this chapter.

1. Tissue management (debridement)

In the context of WBP, tissue management involves the removal of non-viable tissue—including necrotic tissue, slough and fibrinous material, and exudate (Ayello & Cuddigan 2004). Unlike acute wounds, chronic wounds require regular 'maintenance debridement' to stimulate healing (Hess & Kirsner 2003).

'Unlike acute wounds, chronic wounds require regular "maintenance debridement" to stimulate healing.'

The use of antiseptics (such as sodium hypochlorite) for chemical debridement

Acronym for principles of WBP

This chapter discusses the application of the principles of wound-bed preparation (WBP). These principles can be remembered with the aid of the acronym 'TIME':

- *T* refers to 'tissue management' (debridement);
- *I* refers to 'infection' or 'inflammation';
- *M* refers to 'moisture imbalance'; and
- *E* refers to 'edge of wound'.

is no longer recommended. It can be painful and can cause damage to underlying and surrounding tissue (Leaper 2002). Newer medicated dressings have antimicrobial action, but without cellular toxicity.

The choice of a debriding method depends on many factors—including the patient's vascular status, the skill of the clinician, patient preference, wound condition, and treatment goal.

There are various methods of debridement. These include:

- biosurgical debridement;
- enzymatic debridement;
- autolytic debridement;
- mechanical debridement; and
- sharp (surgical) debridement.

Each of these is discussed below.

Biosurgical debridement

Larval (or maggot) therapy has become accepted in several countries, including the USA and the UK. It is an old therapy that declined in popularity with the development of antibiotics. However, in view of the emergence of antibiotic-resistant organisms, there has been renewed interest in this form of debridement.

Larval therapy debrides wounds, controls odour, and has antimicrobial activity. The larvae secrete proteolytic enzymes that liquefy

Methods of debridement

The following five methods of debridement are discussed in this portion of the text:

- biosurgical debridement;
- enzymatic debridement;
- autolytic debridement;
- mechanical debridement; and
- sharp (surgical) debridement.

the non-viable tissue on which the larvae feed. The antimicrobial activity is due to ingestion of bacteria and changes in wound pH. Larvae are also thought to promote healing through fibroblast activation (LarvE 2003).

Larval therapy has traditionally been used when other methods of debridement have failed or when sharp debridement is contraindicated. This form of debridement can also be used as a secondary method—such as after sharp surgical debridement or before skin grafting. Larvae can be used in conjunction with systemic antibiotics, and do not have to be removed for radiological investigations.

'Education of the patient is required before proceeding with any form of debridement, and informed written consent should be obtained.'

No significant side-effects have been reported, although susceptible patients can have allergic reactions—such as contact dermatitis and angioedema (Hess & Kirsner 2003). Some patients complain of discomfort (due to change in pH), aesthetic concerns, or a 'crawling feeling'.

Larval therapy is contraindicated for exposed blood vessels and wounds involving major organs (Hess & Kirsner 2003).

Education of the patient is required before proceeding with this therapy (or any form of debridement), and informed written consent should be obtained. To protect the peri-wound area, a hydrocolloid dressing is applied. To prevent migration of the larvae, the wound is covered with a fine nylon net and secured with tape. An absorbent dressing is then applied, and changed as necessary. It is important that enough moisture is present at the wound bed to prevent the larvae from drying out, but there should not be excessive moisture (which can kill the larvae).

The larvae should be changed approximately twice a week. Larvae should be physically removed, counted, and the wound irrigated with warm normal saline. Larval therapy continues until healthy granulation is present.

Enzymatic debridement

The second method of debridement listed on page 92 was *enzymatic debridement*. Manufactured enzymes can be topically applied to a wound to assist the enzymes in the wound to dissolve non-viable tissue in the wound bed. Commercial products that have been developed include:

- bacterial collagenase;
- papain–urea;
- fibrinolysin–DNAse;
- trypsin;
- streptokinase–streptodornase; and
- subtilisin.

These products are not available in all countries, and have varying degrees of popularity (Enoch & Harding 2003). *Bacterial collagenase* is favoured because: (i) it is selective in digesting and removing only devitalised tissue; (ii) it produces less pain; and (iii) it is thought to stimulate healing. This enzyme specifically attacks and breaks down collagen. The *papain–urea combination* is a non-selective fast-acting preparation that breaks down fibrinous material in devitalised tissue. There is a greater inflammatory response with this enzyme preparation, and it can cause increased exudate and pain.

Enzymatic debridement is utilised in non-infected wounds if conservative sharp wound-debridement skills are not available or if surgical debridement would not be tolerated.

The manufacturer's instructions should be followed. Each enzyme product has specific requirements in terms of wound environment and application. In particular, all enzymes have a specific wound pH for optimal activity. The wound pH can be determined with a litmus strip. Products such as silver, hydrogen peroxide, zinc, and acidic or alkaline solutions can inactivate enzymes.

Enzymatic debridement should not be used in infected wounds or on important viable tissues (for example, tendons and blood vessels). Treatment should be discontinued when the wound is clean.

'Enzymatic debridement should not be used in infected wounds or on important viable tissues.'

In dry necrotic wounds, the eschar should be scored to allow the enzyme to penetrate through to the wound base more quickly. Scoring requires a sharp instrument (such as a scalpel), and involves cutting almost to the depth of the eschar. Care should be taken not to cut into the wound base. Once the necrotic tissue begins to lift away from the edges, conservative sharp debridement (see this chapter, page 97) can be used to hasten the debriding process. Enzymes or autolytic debridement can then be resumed as required. Dressings depend on the manufacturers' guidelines.

Autolytic debridement

The third method of debridement listed on page 92 was *autolytic debridement*. Autolytic debridement encourages naturally occurring wound enzymes to debride a wound selectively (Ramundo & Wells 2000). This method of debridement is a slower method of debridement, but it is easy and painless. Autolytic debridement is indicated for patients when other methods of debridement might not be tolerated, or in conjunction with other debridement methods.

'Autolytic debridement encourages naturally occurring wound enzymes to debride a wound selectively.'

Wounds naturally produce enzymes to break down non-viable tissue. However, if a wound is allowed to dry out, or does not produce enough of its own moisture, debridement will not occur. The use of occlusive, semi-occlusive, moisture-retentive, and moisture-donating dressings provides an environment that facilitates softening, liquefaction, and separation of non-viable tissue.

Honey is gaining popularity because it debrides quickly, deodorises the wound, and has antimicrobial activity (Enoch & Harding 2003). This method can be painful, and requires a medical honey or a pasteurised honey.

The wound and peri-wound area must be monitored for signs of infection and maceration. If the wound is infected, a quicker debridement method should be implemented, and the infection treated.

'Honey debrides quickly, deodorises the wound, and has antimicrobial activity.'

The most commonly used dressings for autolytic debridement include transparent films, hydrogels, hydrocolloids, alginates, and hydrofibre dressings. It is important to select a dressing that is appropriate to the wound condition, the level of exudate, and size of wound. The frequency of dressing changes depends on the dressing type and the level of exudate.

Mechanical debridement

The fourth method of debridement listed on page 92 was *mechanical debridement*. Mechanical debridement requires the use of physical force to remove non-viable or contaminated tissue. It produces rapid debridement, but is non-selective and can cause pain.

As with all forms of debridement, mechanical debridement should be discontinued when the wound is clean and granulation is evident. Nurses using these therapies should remember to wear protective eyewear and clothing. Care should be taken to prevent cross-contamination and aerosolisation.

These forms of debridement are labour-intensive due to frequency of treatment. They can be painful.

Mechanical debridement includes:

- whirlpool therapy;
- wet-to-dry dressings; and
- high-pressure irrigation.

Each of these is discussed below.

Whirlpool therapy

Whirlpool therapy is popular in the USA. It is effective in softening and loosening debris and non-viable tissue. Whirlpool therapy requires a tank with water jets and lifting devices to lower the patient, or rails so that the patient can enter safely. Normal tap water is usually employed, but antiseptics are often added (which can also affect healing).

Whirlpool therapy is thought to work through hydration and the vigorous action of the jets (Ramundo & Wells 2000). This form of debridement is indicated for wounds of large surface area located in an anatomical area that can be immersed.

Whirlpool therapy should be used cautiously in patients with decreased sensation.

Wet-to-dry dressings

Wet-to-dry dressings involve the application of moistened gauze, and allowing it to dry. Woven cotton gauze should be moistened, but not saturated. Normal saline is usually employed. The dressing is placed in the wound so that it contacts the entire wound bed, but not the surrounding skin. A dry secondary dressing is then applied and the dressing is allowed to dry out. The gauze is then removed dry—thus pulling gauze and the attached tissue from the wound. This should be done approximately three times a day. The patient might require premedication before the dressing change.

'Wet-to-dry dressings are used for heavily contaminated wounds with devitalised tissue. Wounds with heavy exudate are not suitable.'

Wet-to-dry dressings are used for heavily contaminated wounds with devitalised tissue. Wounds with heavy exudate are not suitable for wet-to-dry dressings because heavy exudate prevents the 'drying-out' phase.

This form of debridement is commonly used, but it is controversial. It can cause discomfort. Moistening the gauze before removal decreases the discomfort, but defeats the purpose. Autolytic debridement is preferable because it is painless, selective, and easy.

High-pressure irrigation

Irrigation is indicated for visually contaminated wounds. High-pressure irrigation involves the application of pressurised fluid to the wound base. This can be continuous high pressure, or pulsatile lavage. Irrigation pressures of 8–15 pounds per square inch (approx. 400–800 mm Hg) are directed to the contaminated or necrotic tissue. This provides adequate pressure to dislodge and wash away debris and bacteria. If irrigating pressure is too high it can cause debris and organisms to be driven into the deeper tissues.

'Irrigation is indicated for visually contaminated wounds.'

High-pressure irrigation requires a 35-mL syringe and a 19-gauge drawing-up needle or angiocatheter. Warm normal saline is used. Commercially available products provide pulsatile high-pressure irrigation and have the convenience of adjustable pressure levels combined with suction.

Safety and infection-control principles should be strictly followed.

Sharp (surgical) debridement

The fifth method of debridement listed on page 92 was *sharp (surgical) debridement*. Sharp debridement diminishes the bacterial burden, the necrotic burden, and the cellular burden.

Conservative sharp wound debridement is a quick and selective method of debridement that involves removal of loose, non-adherent, non-viable tissue. However, it is not aggressive enough to expose viable tissue (Ramundo & Wells 2000). Conservative sharp debridement is used for 'maintenance debridement'. It might be undertaken over days to weeks until the debridement goal has been achieved. Non-medical health professionals who have been adequately trained and educated in this technique frequently perform this method of debridement.

'Conservative sharp wound debridement is a quick and selective method that involves removal of loose, non-adherent, non-viable tissue.'

More aggressive surgical debridement can be used to remove large amounts of necrotic tissue quickly. This procedure is usually performed by medical practitioners in sterile environments.

Before surgical debridement is undertaken, patients should be assessed for clotting disorders—which might be due to medications or disease. Infected wounds and patients who are immunocompromised might require systemic antibiotics and medicated dressings to reduce bacterial load and dissemination of bacteria. Sharp debridement might require analgesia and either local or general anaesthetic.

Sharp debridement should not be undertaken unless:

- the clinician performing the debridement has been educated and credentialled in debridement technique;
- the patient has provided informed consent (including agreement on what is to be debrided and when to stop); and
- adequate sterile supplies are available.

Conservative sharp debridement should not be undertaken on fungating or malignant wounds. It should also not be used in wounds on the hands and face (Fairbairn et al. 2002).

Surgical debridement usually requires admission to a surgical department where a team provides care before, during, and after the procedure.

2. Infection

The second of the WBP principles listed on page 90 (using the acronym 'TIME') was *infection*. It is generally accepted that all chronic wounds contain bacteria. The bacterial load of a wound can be divided into four categories:

- *contamination:* the presence of non-multiplying microorganisms in a wound;
- *colonisation:* the presence of multiplying microorganisms in a wound, but without a host response (no visible change); colonisation by itself is not enough to impair healing;

- *critical colonisation:* the presence of microorganisms that are multiplying to the degree that healing is impaired, but tissue damage has not occurred (Edwards & Harding 2004); signs and symptoms are limited and do not involve surrounding tissue;
- *infection:* the presence of multiplying organisms with visible changes due to tissue damage; the infection can be local (including cellulitis) or systemic (sepsis).

Disease process and medications can diminish a normal inflammatory response. The classic signs and symptoms of infection might not therefore be apparent. Awareness of the secondary signs of infection can assist in detecting and diagnosing a wound infection. The Box below lists the classic and secondary signs and symptoms of a wound infection.

Signs and symptoms of infection

Classic signs and symptoms
- increased exudate (or change in exudate)
- pain (or change in sensation) in wound area
- new (or increased) erythema
- increased temperature of peri-wound area
- odour (wound or exudate)

Secondary signs
- non-healing wound
- unhealthy granulation (friable, pale hypergranulation)
- increased slough
- increasing wound size
- new areas of breakdown
- pocketing or undermining of wound edges, or bridging of tissue

If there are signs and symptoms of infection present, antibiotics can be started empirically. However, before commencing antibiotics it is useful to obtain a wound swab for microscopy and culture. When the results become available, the sensitivity or resistance of the organisms to the antibiotics can be assessed.

To obtain a wound swab for culture, the wound should first be cleansed with normal saline. Superficial debridement can be undertaken. The swab should be taken from a section of granulation tissue (viable tissue) with the most obvious signs of infection. The specimen should be kept in a refrigerator if a delay is expected (but no more than 24 hours). Fresh wound fluid can be aspirated for microbiological testing. Swabs should not be taken from areas of pus, slough, or surrounding skin. If the wound is dry, the swab can be moistened with sterile normal saline (Sibbald et al. 2003).

'Because of the rising incidence of bacterial resistance, antibiotics are no longer used routinely as first-line management in all infections.'

Antibiotics are commonly used to treat wounds with high levels of bacteria. However, because of the rising incidence of bacterial resistance, antibiotics are no longer used routinely as first-line management in all infections. Other treatment methods include: (i) improving the general health of the patient; (ii) debridement; (iii) cleansing the wound; (iv) slow-release antiseptics; and (v) topical antimicrobial dressings.

Two examples of slow-release antiseptic/antimicrobial agents are cadexomer-iodine and nanocrystalline silver. Silver is also available in other dressings—such as foams, hydrocolloids, alginates, and films (Schultz et al. 2003).

Topical antimicrobials are appropriate for superficial and local infections. However, resistance can develop if they are used on a long-term basis.

Systemic antibiotics are still required for active systemic and deep-tissue infections.

3. Moisture imbalance

The third of the WBP principles listed on page 90 (using the acronym 'TIME') was *moisture imbalance*. Chronic wound fluid is different from acute wound fluid, and a build-up of exudate can be a factor in delayed healing. Maintaining the moisture balance in a wound is a key component of wound-bed preparation.

Desiccation (drying out) of a wound bed prevents migration and activity of epidermal cells; in contrast, excessive fluid can cause maceration leading to erosion of the wound edges. The Box below provides a list of the common causes of chronic wounds being too dry or too moist.

Causes of dry and moist wounds

Causes of excessive wound dryness

If a wound is too dry it might be due to:

- topical mismanagement (that is, the wrong dressing);
- a poorly vascularised wound bed;
- necrotic tissue; or
- the wound being left exposed for too long.

Causes of excessive wound moisture

If a wound is too moist it might be due to:

- topical mismanagement (that is, the wrong dressing);
- lack of compression (in the case of a venous ulcer);
- chronic inflammation;
- a foreign body in the wound (for example, suture material); or
- an underlying medical condition.

Moisture balance can be maintained by applying the correct dressing for the level of exudate and condition of the wound. This requires accurate identification of wound aetiology and assessment of the wound characteristics.

A simple and effective way to assist in moisture balance is to cleanse the wound bed with water or normal saline. This removes debris and static fluid. Excessive moisture can also be treated with topical therapy and ostomy appliances.

Protection of the peri-wound area can be accomplished with the application of barrier ointments or wipes.

4. Management of the edge of the wound

The fourth of the WBP principles listed on page 90 (using the acronym 'TIME') was *edge of wound*.

Non-advancing wound edges can be associated with:

- hyperproliferation of cells at the wound edges;
- lack of migration across granulation tissue;
- senescent cells; and
- undermining of wound edges.

Epidermal tissue at the wound edges should not be confused with maceration. Epidermal tissue is pale and slightly opaque.

Undermining is commonly found in pressure ulcers in which shear and infection are contributing factors. Undermining can be assessed and documented by gently inserting a cotton-tip 'bud' into the wound edges, and then placing it next to a ruler for measurement.

'The wound edges and peri-wound area reflect the health of the wound, and should be continually assessed and documented.'

The wound edges and peri-wound area reflect the health of the wound, and should be continually assessed and documented.

Complications in WBP

Having considered the application of the four main principles of WBP (utilising the acronym 'TIME'), two important complications in WBP deserve consideration. These are:

- osteomyelitis; and
- hypergranulation.

Osteomyelitis

Osteomyelitis can occur in any wound in which bone is exposed to infection—including traumatic wounds and pressure ulcers. Particular risk factors include:

- diabetes mellitus;
- peripheral neuropathy;

- peripheral vascular disease;
- poor glycaemic control in diabetes;
- impaired skin integrity;
- foot deformity;
- advanced age; and
- exposed bone in the wound.

A simple but useful test to detect possible bone involvement is to probe the wound with a metal probe. If bone is felt or visualised, further investigations should be undertaken to determine if osteomyelitis is present (Grayson et al. 1995). These investigations can include a plain X-ray, magnetic-resonance imaging (MRI), C-reactive protein (CRP), erythrocyte sedimentation rate (ESR), and white cell count (WCC). Wound and bone cultures should be obtained if appropriate.

Antibiotics appropriate to the patient, clinical presentation, and cultures should be administered and continued as required.

Hypergranulation

In normal healing, granulation formation should decrease as it fills the wound bed. Hypergranulation ('proud flesh') occurs when the wound environment is out of balance—due to infection, occlusive dressing, or an imbalance of collagen synthesis and lysis.

A wound will not heal if hypergranulation tissue is present. Epithelial cells will not migrate across this engorged tissue.

Treatment depends on the clinical presentation and patient preference. Treatment options include:

- silver nitrate sticks;
- local compression;
- change of dressing to foams or alginates;
- cutting the hypergranulation tissue with a scalpel or scissors;
- medicated dressings (for example, silver or cadexomer-iodine);
- systemic antibiotics and/or topical management; and
- topical steroids.

Conclusion

For many years acute wound-healing models have been used to treat chronic wounds. However, the chronic wound environment is physiologically different from that of acute wounds. A knowledge of wound-bed preparation can assist nurses to manage chronic wounds effectively.

'The principles of WBP allow nurses to implement strategies that will assist the person with a chronic wound to achieve optimal outcomes.'

The principles of WBP allow nurses to implement strategies that will assist the person with a chronic wound to achieve optimal outcomes.

Chapter 7
Nutrition and Healing
Linda Kilworth

Introduction

Nutrition and hydration are important factors in wound management. Healing is enhanced by the provision of all nutrients required for tissue restoration and strengthening of the immune system. Conversely, insufficient energy, protein, vitamins, minerals, and water are all associated with skin breakdown and delayed healing (Ferguson et al. 2000).

Anabolic and catabolic processes

Anabolism is the process of construction and regeneration, whereas catabolism is the dismantling and breaking-down of structures. In a healthy person, the two processes work synergistically.

People with chronic wounds are often catabolic and require extra energy (kilojoules) and protein. In many cases it is difficult to know whether the weight loss and malnutrition lead to skin breakdown, or whether the presence of a wound contributes to weight loss and malnutrition. Whatever the mechanism, people with wounds require good nutrition and adequate energy intake.

Weight loss, particularly if it is involuntary, can have a deleterious effect on wound healing. Weight loss of as little as 5% can be significant—especially in the very young or very old.

Framework of the chapter
This chapter discusses nutrition and healing under the following headings:
- anabolic and catabolic processes (page 105);
- general nutritional assessment (this page);
- nutritional requirements for wound healing (page 110);
- goals of nutritional intervention (page 113); and
- summary of recommendations (page 119).

General nutritional assessment

A general nutrition-care plan should consider all aspects of a person's needs and preferences. This includes consideration of:
- the person's ability to eat and drink;
- food preferences;
- appetite;
- food textures;
- hydration;
- elimination; and
- measurable parameters.

Each of these is considered below.

Ability to eat and drink

Nurses and dietitians should check for medical conditions that might affect a person's ability to eat and drink. These include such factors as dysphagia (swallowing difficulties), cognitive impairment, and dietary restrictions. Dietary restrictions might be required for various medical conditions (such as diabetes) or might be self-imposed.

General nutritional assessment

This section of the chapter discusses the following aspects of general nutritional assessment:

- the person's ability to eat and drink;
- food preferences;
- appetite;
- food textures;
- hydration;
- elimination; and
- measurable parameters.

Food preferences

People often have personal likes and dislikes with respect to food, and these should be taken into account—especially if appetite is poor. It might be necessary to consider alternatives that appeal to the person.

Appetite

To facilitate food intake, meal plans should be individualised to suit the person's needs. Some people prefer large servings at meals, whereas others prefer small frequent meals. Some people prefer a large cooked breakfast, whereas others prefer a 'continental style' breakfast. Some people are drowsy during the day, but active at night or in the early hours of the morning—and consume more food during their 'active' times. Every person is an individual, and this should be taken into account when planning a food plan to optimise nutrition.

'Every person is an individual, and this should be taken into account when planning a food plan to optimise nutrition.'

Food textures

People who are receiving texture-modified foods (such as minced or puréed meals) are likely to consume fewer kilojoules. In addition, people who are receiving texture-modified diets are not likely to be offered mid-meal snacks. These diets are often supplemented with a nutritious drink and little else. Adding more high-energy food at mealtimes, rather than supplementation at other times, can be beneficial.

In institutional settings, time and staffing issues in food service can cause difficulties. If so, there are many commercially available foods available to add energy—such as yoghurt, puréed fruit, custards, and cheesecakes.

Hydration

Dehydration can affect a person's appetite, increase confusion, and interfere with elimination. Varying the fluid (rather than offering only water) can make fluids more palatable.

High-energy fluids are preferred for people who are underweight whereas low-energy fluids are preferred for those who are overweight.

Elimination

Constipation and diarrhoea both affect appetite. Assessment of current bowel habits is necessary to determine the type of nutritional intervention required. Increasing fibre and fluids might be necessary.

Measurable parameters

Certain measurable factors should be monitored. These include:

- weight, height, and body mass index;
- serum albumin; and
- serum cholesterol.

Weight, height, and body mass index

Weight should be measured when the person is first seen, and checked at monthly intervals thereafter. This should be recorded on a graph, so that a visual picture of weight trends can be identified.

A loss of 5% of normal body weight is considered significant. For example, if a person has a usual weight of 50 kg, a weight loss of 2.5 kg is considered significant.

Height should also be measured when the person is first seen. This can then be used, in association with weight, to calculate the person's body mass index (BMI). BMI is calculated according to the following formula (with weight being measured in kilograms and height in metres):

$$BMI = weight/height^2$$

For example, using the above formula, a person with a height of 2 metres who weighed 50 kilograms would have a BMI of:

$$50/2^2 = 50/4 = 12.5$$

This person would therefore have a BMI of 12.5 kg/m^2.

The significance of various BMIs is shown in Table 7.1 (below). In the example given above, the person with a calculated BMI of 12.5 would therefore be considered underweight.

Table 7.1 Significance of BMIs
AUTHOR'S PRESENTATION; REPRODUCED FROM CARMODY & FORSTER (2003)

BMI	Significance
Less than 20	Underweight
20–25	Acceptable weight
25–30	Overweight
Greater than 30	Obese

Serum albumin
Serum albumin provides a useful indication of nutritional status. Albumin levels can drop as a result of protein loss from exudative wounds. In addition, low serum albumin levels (less than 35 g/L) can impair delivery of nutrients to the wound site itself.

Serum cholesterol
A decreased level of cholesterol can predispose to the development of pressure ulcers. Indeed, low levels of cholesterol are a more accurate

predictor of the development of such wounds than low albumin levels (Escott-Stump 1998).

Nutritional requirements for wound healing

Having considered the person's general requirements for a nutrition-care plan, nurses and dietitians should pay special attention to the nutritional requirements for wound healing. This includes consideration of:

- energy;
- protein;
- fluid;
- vitamins A and C;
- zinc; and
- arginine and glutamine.

    Each of these is discussed below.

Energy

It is important to provide sufficient energy to facilitate wound healing. Significant weight loss is associated with poor skin integrity.

There are many ways to estimate energy needs. The Harris Benedict equation is often used by dietitians to establish exact daily energy requirements (Bartlett et al. 1998). This equation uses the basal metabolic rate and an 'activity factor' to determine daily energy needs in terms of kilojoules (or Calories).

'Significant weight loss is associated with poor skin integrity.'

For a less exact estimation, an alternative 'rule-of-thumb' method for determining energy requirements is as follows:

Weight of patient (kg) $\times$ 126 = energy (kJ) required for maintenance of current weight

Weight of patient (kg) $\times$ 147 = energy (kJ) required for weight gain

Nutritional requirements for wound healing

This section of the chapter discusses the following aspects of nutritional requirements for wound healing:

- energy;
- protein;
- fluid;
- vitamins A and C;
- zinc; and
- arginine and glutamine.

Protein

Protein is required for tissue growth and repair. In particular, the nitrogen in protein is required for replication of lymphocytes, fibroblasts, and granulation tissue.

A person's requirements are usually calculated as 1.25–1.5 grams per kilogram of body weight per day (Ferguson et al. 2000). A person who weighs 50 kg therefore requires approximately 62.5 g (50 x 1.25) of protein per day.

It is important to take into account individual medical conditions that can affect a person's protein requirements. For example, some medical conditions (such as kidney disease) require low-protein diets. Higher protein intake might not be suitable in these people.

Fluid

A person's hydration status is important for the maintenance of blood volume and circulation. Total fluid requirements (including fluid from food) can be calculated as 30–35 millilitres per kilogram of body weight per day. Therefore, a person who weighs 50 kg requires approximately 1500 mL (50 x 30) of fluid per day.

Vitamins A and C

Vitamin A is important for proper functioning of the immune system, development of epithelium, and synthesis of collagen. The recommended amount is 1000 micrograms per day for males and 800 micrograms per day for females (Ferguson et al. 2000). Vitamin A is found in coloured vegetables and fruits (such as broccoli, spinach, carrots, squash, sweet potatoes, pumpkin, cantaloupe, and apricots). It is also found in animal sources such as liver, red meat, milk, butter, cheese, and whole eggs.

'Vitamin A is important for proper functioning of the immune system, development of epithelium, and synthesis of collagen.'

Vitamin C is a water-soluble vitamin and antioxidant. It plays a part in collagen synthesis and in stimulating the immune system. The recommended minimum intake is 60 mg per day. Foods high in vitamin C include citrus fruits, strawberries, cranberries, tomatoes, peppers, dark-green leafy vegetables, potatoes, and broccoli. One glass of orange juice provides approximately 120 mg of vitamin C. The recommended daily intake of vitamin C for wound healing is greater than the recommended daily intake for healthy people. An intake of greater than 250 mg is recommended for wound healing.

'The recommended daily intake of vitamin C for wound healing is greater than the recommended daily intake for healthy people.'

Zinc

Zinc is a mineral that plays a part in tissue synthesis and in strengthening the immune system. The recommended amount is 15 mg per day (Ferguson et al. 2000). The best source of zinc is oysters (12 mg per oyster). Liver, red meat, beans, nuts, seeds, and wholegrains are also good sources of zinc.

Arginine and glutamine

Arginine is concentrated in skin and connective tissue and increases collagen deposition (Schmidt 2002). Arginine is also involved in the regulation of nucleic acid synthesis, which is important for cell growth and replication. Arginine thus works at the cellular level to assist healing and stimulate the immune response (Schmidt 2002). Arginine is found in protein-rich foods—such as egg and nuts. Wholegrains are also rich in arginine. There are also commercial supplementary drinks available that are rich in arginine. These are quite palatable and are easier for some people to consume than other sources of arginine.

'Arginine works at the cellular level to assist healing and stimulate the immune response.'

Glutamine is an amino acid that acts as a 'fuel source' for rapidly dividing cells. It therefore has an indirect role in healing. At present, there is no firm evidence that glutamine supplementation is helpful for wound healing, but glutamine is likely to assist in epithelial repair. Glutamine is abundant in all foods, and dietary deficiencies of this amino acid are therefore rare.

'Glutamine is abundant in all foods, and dietary deficiencies of this amino acid are therefore rare.'

Goals of nutritional intervention

The main goals of nutritional intervention for wound healing are:

- to restore normal nutritional status by correcting malnutrition (if present);
- to provide sufficient nutrients to prevent further tissue breakdown;
- to support the immune system to reduce infections; and
- to maintain healthy skin once healing has occurred.

Each of these is discussed in further detail below.

1. Restoration of nutritional status

There are many factors to consider when attempting to restore nutritional status. These include the person's medical condition, the effects of medications, social factors, environmental factors, and functional disabilities. Some people might have previously been on restricted diet— as a result of a pre-existing medical condition (such as diabetes) or by preference (such as vegetarianism).

Goals of nutritional intervention

This section of the chapter discusses the main goals of nutritional intervention. These are:

- to restore normal nutritional status by correcting malnutrition (if present);
- to provide sufficient nutrients to prevent further tissue breakdown;
- to support the immune system to reduce infections; and
- to maintain healthy skin once healing has occurred.

A high-energy, high-protein diet is used, unless contraindicated. Increased energy and protein can be supplied by:

- increased total food and beverage intake;
- oral supplements (with meals or between meals); and
- enteral feeding (via a nasogastric tube or gastrostomy tube).

Each of these is discussed in further detail below.

Increased total food and beverage intake

Total energy can be increased by offering energy-dense food and fluids. If overall food intake is insufficient, all food and beverages should be energy-dense. In terms of fluid intake, milk, milk drinks, food drinks, milky coffee, or juice should therefore be offered—rather than water. Foods with high protein content include cheese, peanut paste, egg, milk powder, milk, soy, and yoghurt.

Offering snacks such as yoghurt, mousse, instant puddings, custards, frozen desserts, cheese and biscuit snacks, and sandwiches increases the nutrient content of the diet.

Table 7.2 (page 115) provides ideas for increasing the energy and protein content of foods. The information in this table might be especially useful for older patients, or those who are unwell.

Table 7.2 Ideas for increasing protein and energy content of foods

AUTHOR'S PRESENTATION

Food or mealtime	Suggestions
Meat, poultry, fish	Blend with gravy or sauce Serve with extra gravy or sauce Add cream, grated cheese, or milk powder to white sauces
Eggs	Add extra yolk to scrambled or soft poached eggs
Nuts and legumes	Add mashed baked beans, lentils, dried peas, or mushy peas to main meal dishes and soups Alternatively, serve as accompaniment to meals
Milk and dairy products	Use full-cream dairy products or milk powder whenever possible Make up fortified milk (100 mL of milk with 1–2 tablespoons of milk powder) and use whenever possible (including in beverages) Milk powder or coconut-milk powder can be added to porridge
Soups	Blend milk (or cream), a raw egg, or grated cheese into home-made or canned soups Add legumes and vegetables to soups
Vegetables	Serve blended (or mashed) with milk, milk powder, cream, extra butter, or cheese Sour cream and margarine added to vegetables adds extra flavour
Cereals	Serve semolina, rolled oats, or cereals softened with milk Add milk powder or coconut-milk powder to boost energy content Serve cereals with milk (or cream) and sugar
Fruit	Offer puréed, mashed, stewed, or soft fresh fruits (banana, pear, pawpaw) Serve with cream, yoghurt, custard, or a milky dessert
Dessert	Custard, ice-cream, creamed rice, blancmange, junket, baked egg custard, milk jelly, mousse, cheesecake, dairy snacks
Mid-meal ideas	Biscuit or wheat breakfast biscuit shake (see Box, page 116) Fruit smoothie Cake or biscuit soaked in milk Bread and butter soaked in milk (or blended)

Biscuit or wheat breakfast biscuit shake

A 'biscuit shake' is an easy way to offer increased energy and protein in the diet. This can be prepared as follows.

Ingredients
- 200 mL whole milk
- 1 tablespoon cream
- 1 tablespoon sugar or honey
- 2–3 wheat breakfast biscuits (or biscuits)

Method
- blend together in mixer;
- add extra milk to reach the desired consistency;
- add extra honey or sugar to taste;
- serve.

Oral supplements

As noted on page 114, the second method of increasing energy and protein in the diet is by providing oral supplements (with meals or between meals). There are many commercial supplements available in various flavours. Alternatively, homemade beverages (such as fruit 'smoothies', malted milks, and warm food drinks) can be offered.

High-protein formulae that provide 1.5–4.0 Calories per mL are commercially available. These are useful for promoting wound healing, although there are some medical contraindications.

'Supplements are not a substitute for normal food.'

It should be noted that supplements are not a substitute for normal food. They are most useful with people who prefer fluids to food. Many people will take supplementary drinks initially, but later refuse them due to taste fatigue. It is important to enhance the flavour using various toppings and fruits. People who dislike drinking too much fluid, but who are eating well, can have a scoop of a commercially available supplement added to porridge, cereal, soups, and sauces.

Med Pass™ type programs can be beneficial. These have energy-dense formulae containing 2–7 Calories per mL of fluid. They can be offered in doses of 60–80 mL several times per day as part of medication rounds. This can contribute a significant energy intake, especially for people who have poor appetites. In institutional settings, the Med Pass™ system relieves food-service staff of responsibility for supplementation, and allows nursing staff to ensure (and document) that the high-energy high-protein supplement is consumed (Chang 1997).

Enteral feeding
A decision to feed a person enterally via a nasogastric tube or gastrostomy tube depends on many factors. These include quality of life, preferences of the person or caregivers, overall status, and life-expectancy.

Enteral feeding can provide the total nutrient intake, or it can supplement oral intake. For supplementation, overnight feeding is preferred—to avoid affecting appetite. Night feeds should be gradually reduced as oral food intake increases.

There is a variety of enteral feeding formulae available. Most standard feeds contain 1 Cal/mL. People with wounds need a high-energy, high-protein formula. There are numerous specialised feeds available, and a dietitian can advise on the correct choice.

2. Providing sufficient nutrients
The second goal of nutritional intervention for people with wounds (page 113) was to provide sufficient nutrients to prevent further tissue breakdown.

Providing an appropriate supplement to people with chronic malnutrition or an obvious vitamin or mineral deficiency is prudent. However, it should be noted that *'Too much of a good thing is not necessarily better.'* supplementation without a deficiency does not increase healing. In other words, 'too much of a good thing is not necessarily better'.

The main nutrients required for wound healing are zinc and vitamins A and C. The Box below provides an example of increasing these nutrients for the different stages of a pressure ulcer.

Nutrients in management of a pressure ulcer

The main nutrients required for wound healing are zinc and vitamins A and C. The following recommendations provide guidance for increasing these healing nutrients in the example of a staged pressure ulcer.

Stage 1 ulcer
- Offer half a cup orange juice or equivalent source of vitamin C (approx. 60 mg vitamin C).

Stage 2 ulcer
- Offer 1 cup orange juice or high-vitamin C beverage (approx 120 mg vitamin C).
- Increase zinc (and protein) with meat (100 g meat contains approx. 3.5 mg zinc).
- Increase zinc (and energy) with a supplementary drink—provides approx. 4.3 mg zinc (and 566 kJ of energy).

Stage 3 ulcer
- Offer one-and-a-half cups of orange juice or food/beverage high in vitamin C.
- Increase protein with 2–3 supplementary drinks (best offered between meals).

Stage 4 ulcer
- Offer one-and-a-half cups of orange juice or food/beverage high in vitamin C.
- Increase protein with 2–3 supplementary drinks and/or consider a higher energy and protein supplement in the form of a Med Pass™ system.

3. Supporting the immune system to reduce infections

The third goal of nutritional intervention for people with wounds (page 113) was to support the immune system to reduce infections. Maintaining a high-energy, high-protein intake supports the immune system. Providing the person with foods that he or she enjoys will enhance this process.

4. Maintaining healthy skin once healing has occurred

To maintain healthy skin once the wound has healed (the fourth objective noted on page 113), an appropriate nutritional intake should be continued.

Monitoring the person's weight on a monthly basis ensures that problems are noted early so that corrective action can be taken. Ensuring that the menu is balanced and provides sufficient variety also assists in maintaining skin integrity.

Fluids should be offered frequently to prevent dehydration. Some people require ongoing supplements or continued enteral feeds.

Summary of recommendations

This chapter has discussed several aspects of nutrition and wound healing. The Box below provides a summary of the dietary recommendations of the chapter.

Summary of recommendations for wound healing

1. Provide a balanced diet by ensuring that the menu is nutritionally sound.
2. Allow for personal preferences and requirements. These include:
   - adhering to individual likes and dislikes, without compromising overall nutrition;
   - taking into account factors producing poor oral intake (such as dysphagia, dementia, and so on);
   - providing foods in an appropriate texture for the person;
   - considering the special needs of people on tube feeds (such as providing high-energy, high-protein enteral formulae).

(continued)

(continued)

3. Provide a high-protein diet with 1.2–1.5 grams of protein per kilogram of body weight. This can be achieved by adding high-protein powders to foods, or by using liquid supplementation.

4. Increase energy intake (if possible and desirable).

5. Supplement the diet with vitamins A and C, and zinc (if a deficiency exists).

6. Consider supplements that are fortified with arginine and glutamine.

7. Ensure that the person is well hydrated (at least 1500 mL fluid daily).

8. Monitor weight monthly and note significant weight changes.

Conclusion

Nutrition is not a guaranteed panacea for the healing of wounds, but can assist in the overall treatment.

There is no direct cause-and-effect relationship between poor nutrition and wound development. However, there is evidence that improving nutritional status can assist in healing.

In practice, wound healing is assisted by improved nutrition and hydration in conjunction with good nursing practice.

Chapter 8
Trauma

Pam Morey

Introduction

Because the skin has a protective function, it is always at risk of physical injury from trauma. Traumatic injuries include contusions, abrasions, tears, incisions, lacerations, punctures and penetrating injuries, thermal wounds, degloving and avulsion injuries, and crush injuries.

'The psychological impact of traumatic injuries should never be overlooked.'

The mechanisms of injury can be broadly categorised as blunt trauma (including shearing and compression injuries) or penetrating trauma (for example, gunshot or stabbing injuries) (Blank-Reid 2004).

The severity of the injury is determined by the depth of injury, damage to underlying structures, and the area of tissue involved.

The role of nurses in response to skin trauma begins with simple first aid, and can progress to more complex wound management. In addition, the psychological impact of traumatic injuries should never be overlooked. Nurses are in a unique position to monitor how their patients are coping, and to offer support as necessary.

This chapter discusses key nursing strategies in the management of traumatic skin wounds according to the framework shown in the Box below.

Framework of the chapter

This chapter discusses the care of traumatic wounds under the following headings:

- First aid (page 122)
- Gunshot wounds (page 125)
- Penetrating injuries (page 126)
- Crush injuries (page 126)
- Degloving injuries (page 128)
- Skin tears (page 128)

First aid

Assessment

First aid might be required in the treatment of a traumatic wound in a variety of settings—including the community, residential care, and hospital. The priorities of first-aid care depend on the severity of injury, but the principles remain the same.

'The priorities of first-aid care depend on the severity of injury, but the principles remain the same.'

Initial assessment of an injured person includes a primary survey to establish priorities of care (Laskowski-Jones 2002; Steffen 2003), followed by a secondary survey and assessment of the wound. Actual treatment then follows.

The general principles of nursing management apply in the first aid of a traumatic wound. The primary assessment and overall safety of the patient must be considered first. This includes isolating the patient from further danger and ensuring that the person's airway, breathing, and circulation are not compromised.

The secondary survey includes identification of obvious injuries and the taking of a history from the person, family, and relevant witness

(Singer, Hollander & Quinn 1997). This includes ascertaining the cause of the injury, co-existing illnesses and other factors that might impair healing, and any allergies (Waller 2004). In the case of a traumatic wound, it is important to establish the person's tetanus-immunisation status because a 'booster' might be required.

'In the case of a traumatic wound, it is important to establish the person's tetanus-immunisation status.'

The location of the wound provides clues as to the possible involvement of underlying structures—including joints, nerves, blood vessels, tendons, bony structures, and organs. Exploration of the wound at the first-aid stage is limited without effective analgesia. If the wound is over a joint, initial immobilisation or splinting of the joint is appropriate.

Amputation

If amputation of a body part has occurred, it is important to recover this part in case it is suitable for later re-attachment. If there is visible dirt or debris on the amputated part, it should be rinsed before being wrapped in a clean towel (moistened with normal saline if available). The body part should then be placed in a clean plastic bag and kept cool or refrigerated (but not frozen). It should accompany the person to the nearest medical facility as soon as possible.

'If amputation of a body part has occurred, it is important to recover this part.'

Foreign bodies

If an object is embedded or impaled in the wound, no attempt should be made to remove it because this can cause bleeding and further tissue damage (Laskowski-Jones 2002). The embedded object should be stabilised with a bulky dressing placed around it.

Haemorrhage

Most traumatic wounds cause some degree of bleeding. The natural haemostatic mechanisms of the body should be facilitated by applying pressure to the area. Firm (but gentle) local pressure should be applied by covering the wound with a clean pad and manually applying pressure (Pignone & Levin 2002).

If sustained pressure is required to arrest bleeding, local compression can be applied with a pad (or bolster) and bandaging (or taping). If circumferential pressure is applied to a limb, it is important to observe the distal circulation to ensure that this is not compromised. In the case of a wound on a limb, elevation of the limb will also help to reduce bleeding.

'If circumferential pressure is applied to a limb, it is important to observe the distal circulation.'

If the person takes anticoagulant or anti-platelet medication (such as warfarin or aspirin), this will increase the risk of bleeding.

Cleansing

Once the bleeding has stopped, the wound should be cleaned—provided that this is unlikely to provoke further bleeding. Proper cleansing reduces bacterial contamination and removes loose debris in the wound—thereby minimising the likelihood of infection (Waller 2004).

The choice of cleansing agents is determined by such factors as whether the wound is dirty and contaminated, the depth of injury, involvement of other organs, the environment in which the injury has occurred, the immune status of the person, and the availability of products (AWMA 2002).

'Normal saline … is economical, effective, and non-toxic to tissue.'

Ideally, normal saline should be used because this is economical, effective, and non-toxic to tissue (Singer, Hollander & Quinn 1997). In the absence of sterile wound-cleansers, clean (drinking-quality) water can be used.

The wound should be irrigated or flushed well. A syringe and blunt large-bore needle provides sufficient pressure to effect the removal of loose debris and bacteria. Alternatively, running water from a tap can be used. In dirty, heavily contaminated wounds, it might be appropriate to consider the use of an antiseptic.

In addition to cleaning the wound, the surrounding skin should be washed and dried (Pignone & Levin 2002). If the wound is in a hairy location, it might be necessary to clip the hair (Singer, Hollander & Quinn 1997.

Dressings

In a minor injury, a dressing might be used to cover the wound. The choice of dressings is discussed in more detail in Chapter 4, 'Dressings', page 51.

Some wounds require primary closure through the use of skin-closure strips, tissue adhesives, or sutures. Others require an interim dressing until surgical treatment is arranged. Others are left to heal by secondary intention with ongoing dressings.

'Even with initial first aid, it is important to remember the principles of moist wound-healing.'

Even with initial first aid, it is important to remember the principles of moist wound-healing, and the risk of further trauma should always be minimised when applying dressings.

Gunshot wounds

Gunshot wounds can be either *penetrating* (with entry, but no exit) or *perforating* (in which there is an entry wound *and* an exit wound) (Silva 1999).

Different bullets have different capacities to cause damage. The type of bullet, and how the bullet interacts with the tissue it encounters, determine the degree of injury. Bullets cause two types of initial injury— 'crush' injuries and 'stretch' injuries (Silva 1999). The tissue is crushed by the penetrating projectile and/or displaced as the projectile travels through the tissue.

Gunshot wounds usually require surgery to debride or repair damaged tissue, although some pellets or fragments can be left in situ if their removal would be likely to cause more problems than would be solved by their removal. In view of the tissue damage often associated with gunshot wounds, antibiotic cover is usually required to prevent infection.

Wound care is based on local management of the particular wound involved. It might include cleansing, drainage, and exudate management.

As with all traumatic injuries, the psychological impact of a gunshot wound should not be overlooked. Counselling and debriefing might be required. Nurses are in a unique position to monitor how individuals are coping, and to offer psychological support as necessary.

Penetrating injuries

The depth, degree of injury, and volume of bleeding from penetrating wounds (such as stabbing wounds) is determined by the type of stabbing implement that inflicts the wound.

Penetrating injuries that have embedded objects usually require a surgical procedure to effect removal without further trauma—particularly if the object is jagged.

Penetrating injuries often require surgical exploration and repair of underlying structures or organs.

Crush injuries

Crush injuries occur when tissue is compressed between two solid objects. This leads to underlying skin and muscle damage—with or without bony fractures. The skin might be contused or necrotic, and it can take several days before the viability of tissue becomes apparent.

'It can take several days before the viability of tissue becomes apparent.'

Significant crush injuries to limbs have a high likelihood of 'compartment syndrome'—which describes damage to nerves, blood vessels, and muscles within the enclosed spaces formed by fascial layers (Kurt et al. 2003). Crush injuries involving limbs should therefore be observed regularly and frequently for the '6Ps'—pain, pallor, paraesthesia, paralysis, pulselessness, and poikilothermy (coldness). Compartment syndrome requires urgent surgical intervention with fasciotomy to avoid permanent damage to the limb.

'6Ps' and compartment syndrome

Crush injuries involving limbs are liable to develop compartment syndrome. Limbs should be observed carefully for the '6Ps':

- pain;
- pallor;
- paraesthesia;
- paralysis;
- pulselessness; and
- poikilothermy (coldness).

Other complications of major crush injury can include (Kurt et al. 2003):

- rhabdomyolysis—breakdown of muscle fibres resulting in the release of muscle-fibre contents (some of which are toxic to the kidneys) into the circulation;
- myonecrosis—death of muscle tissue;
- myoglobinuria—passage of myoglobulin (muscle protein) in the urine, which can be associated with renal failure;
- hyperkalaemia—raised serum potassium levels;
- metabolic acidosis;
- coagulation defects;
- acute renal failure; and
- shock.

Infection is also a risk, and antibiotics are usually prescribed.

Nursing management is targeted at delivering adequate fluid replacement. Aggressive fluid replacement and the promotion of diuresis are required in major crush injuries. Subsequent monitoring of urinary output should be performed to evaluate renal function.

Pain management and the general monitoring of vital signs are both important aspects of nursing care in crush injuries.

Appropriate wound management is necessary—whether this be dealing with a post-surgical wound (following fasciotomy or debridement of non-viable tissue) or caring for a lesser crush injury (that does not require surgery). In crush injuries of a limb or a digit, it is important to elevate the part to prevent (or reduce) swelling.

'In crush injuries of a limb or a digit, it is important to elevate the part to prevent (or reduce) swelling.'

Degloving injuries

Degloving injuries involve the removal of tissue from a limb or digit as if removing a glove. It is not uncommon for a ring worn on a finger to become caught in machinery and cause this type of injury.

Degloving injuries can be complete or partial—depending on whether the tissue is stripped off completely or has a remnant attached (McGregor 1990). The underlying structure of bone and tendon is often left intact. However, nerves and vessels are likely to be damaged in degloving injuries.

'Nerves and vessels are likely to be damaged in degloving injuries.'

First aid is important (see above, page 122), and subsequent surgical review is required to assess the viability of the degloved tissue. It is common for this type of injury to be repaired by a skin graft or a flap—depending on the extent of the injury. Sometimes the detached tissue can be revascularised and replaced (McGregor 1990).

Skin tears

A skin tear can be defined as (Payne & Martin 1990):

> … a traumatic wound that occurs principally on the extremities of older adults as a result of friction alone, or shearing and friction forces, which separate the epidermis from the dermis (partial-thickness wound) or which separate both the epidermis and dermis from underlying structures (full-thickness wound).

Skin tears can be classified into three categories, as shown in Table 8.1 (page 129).

Table 8.1 Classification of skin-tear wounds

AUTHOR'S PRESENTATION ADAPTED FROM PAYNE & MARTIN (1993)

Category	Subcategory	Description
Category I		those without tissue loss (deficit of 1 mm or less)
	Ia	linear-type
	Ib	flap-type
Category II		variable tissue loss
	IIa	scanty tissue loss (equal to or less than 25%)
	IIb	moderate tissue loss (more than 25%)
Category III		complete tissue loss

Skin tears are a common problem in the elderly in residential care, domiciliary care, and tertiary care. Skin tears are especially prevalent in older people because of age-related skin changes and various disease processes that predispose to injury. Those at particular risk are frail, elderly females with dementia (or impaired cognition), those who are dependent on others for activities of daily living, and those who are nutritionally compromised (McGough-Csarny & Kopac 1998; Payne & Martin 1990; White, Karam & Cowell 1994).

'Skin tears are especially prevalent in older people because of age-related skin changes and various disease processes that predispose to injury.'

Initial management focuses on:

- haemostasis and wound cleansing;
- preservation of skin flap (if present);

- promotion of moist wound-healing;
- prevention of infection; and
- protection from further injury.

  Each of these is discussed below.

Haemostasis and wound cleansing

Haemostasis can be achieved by applying gentle pressure or by using a calcium alginate dressing. On occasions, a local pressure dressing might be required—particularly if the person is taking anticoagulant or anti-platelet medication.

'Cleansing of the wound with normal saline is recommended.'

Cleansing of the wound with normal saline is recommended—especially if there is blood or crusting present (Cuzzell 2002). If the wound is dirty or contaminated, an antiseptic might be used to wash the wound. It should then be rinsed with normal saline (Templeton 2003).

Preservation of skin flap

The wound bed and underside of the skin flap (if present) should be cleaned, and any debris or clot should be removed. Ragged edges might need to be trimmed.

'The skin flap can be gently realigned without too much tension.'

The skin flap can then be gently realigned without too much tension using fine metal forceps or moistened cotton tips. The flap should be stabilised and secured with skin-closure strips or a securing dressing (for example, silicone-coated mesh or foam).

Flap-type skin tears are often treated in the same manner as a skin graft, and in these circumstances, the principles of graft care apply (Cuzzell 2002; O'Regan 2002).

Promotion of moist wound healing

The chosen dressing should allow any skin deficit to remain moist while preventing any trauma or maceration to any residual skin flap.

The characteristics of the skin tear influence the choice of product. Dressing alternatives include hydrogels, alginates, tulle gras, foams, hydrocolloids, polyurethane transparent films, skin-closure strips, silicone-coated dressings, and low-adherent dressings.

Prevention of infection

Nurses should endeavour to maintain an aseptic technique when treating the injury. However, this depends on the setting and available resources. People who are at risk (for example, immunocompromised individuals) might require prophylactic antimicrobial dressings—especially if any systemic infection is present.

Protection from further injury

Protection from further injury includes the use of atraumatic dressings, minimal use of adhesive products, and general strategies to prevent further injury.

Special care must be taken with the use of adhesives on the skin. If they must be used, adhesive solvents are advised to assist removal without trauma (Meulenieire 2003). Cohesive, tubular, and crêpe bandages are alternative means of securing the dressing (Cuzzell 2002).

'Special care must be taken with the use of adhesives on the skin.'

It is important to identify and control risk factors—through management of disease processes, care with drug therapy, and modification of the physical environment to prevent injury (Everett & Powell 1994). Prevention of skin tears also requires education of staff and susceptible individuals (and their families) on the risk of injury and strategies to minimise the harm.

Conclusion

Traumatic wounds are very common, and pose challenges to clinicians because they occur suddenly and unexpectedly. Although most traumatic injuries are minor, others require surgery and, perhaps, hospitalisation.

The general principles of wound care apply. An understanding of the mechanism of injury, the structures involved, and the body's response to trauma allows nurses to plan and deliver appropriate wound care to enhance healing.

Nurses have a key role in both the initial management of a traumatic wound and in the subsequent care until the wound is healed. At all times, it is essential to explain aspects of care to patients, and to reassure and support people who have a traumatic injury.

Chapter 9

Reconstructive Techniques

Pam Morey

Introduction

Reconstructive techniques are required in wound management if there is significant tissue loss as a result of injury or surgery. A stepwise approach is appropriate—beginning with the simplest option and working up to more complex procedures. Depending on the person, the injury, and available resources, these stepwise options include suturing, skin grafting, and a variety of skin flaps.

'Aesthetic and functional outcomes are important in deciding on an appropriate procedure.'

Aesthetic and functional outcomes are important in deciding on an appropriate procedure. The final appearance of the wound and the durability of the tissue used to cover the wound defect are the main considerations (Clamon & Netscher 1994). Other factors to consider include the rate of healing, cost-effectiveness, and the technical complexity of the procedure being contemplated (Kane 1997).

Other technologies—such as topical negative pressure therapy (TNPT)—can be considered as an alternative to surgery, or as an adjunct to surgery and conventional wound-care techniques.

The nurses' role is very important in the care of patients undergoing these procedures. Indeed these procedures might be nurse-initiated in some instances of suturing or TNPT.

Reconstructive techniques

This chapter discusses reconstructive techniques under the following headings:

- Reconstructive ladder (page 134)
- Suturing and wound closure (page 134)
- Skin grafts (page 135)
- Flaps (page 139)
- Topical negative pressure therapy (page 142)

Reconstructive ladder

Reconstructive options can be considered as a 'ladder' with steps of increasing complexity. By tradition, the 'reconstructive ladder' begins with healing of a wound by *non-surgical means*—that is, healing by secondary intention. This then 'steps up' to *suturing* of the wound (healing by primary intention), followed by *skin grafting, local flaps, distant flaps*, and *microvascular free tissue transfer* (Clamon & Netscher 1994; Kane 1997).

'Reconstructive options can be considered as a 'ladder' with steps of increasing complexity.'

Each option is more complex than the preceding one. The choice is made in accordance with what is likely to achieve a suitable outcome for the person.

It is postulated that TNPT might, in fact, reduce the complexity of reconstruction required (Banwell & Teot 2003).

Suturing and wound closure

Sutured wounds are common. Whether they are working in a general practice, a hospital emergency department, or a surgical ward, nurses are almost certain to care for people with sutured wounds.

Materials and methods

A number of methods and materials can be employed to suture a wound—including the use of tissue staplers. Tissue adhesives have also become popular because they do not require local anaesthesia and follow-up removal of sutures (Maksud-Sagrillo & Mooney 1999).

Dressings

It is common for the sutured or stapled wound to be covered with an 'island-type' dressing with a central low-adherent pad and an adhesive retention or film dressing. This can stay in place until the wound ceases to produce exudate, unites, and epithelialises—at which time the dressing can be left off.

In some instances, especially on the face, the sutured wound might be left exposed. In these cases it is important to perform suture care, or cleansing, to remove exudate—thereby preventing crusting and minimising the risk of infection and subsequent scarring.

Removal of sutures or staples

Removal of sutures or staples varies—according to the person's own healing rate, the anatomical location of the wound, and the tension on the wound itself. It is important that the wound be assessed before removal of sutures to ensure that healing is complete, and to note the suturing technique that has been employed.

The removal technique varies—depending on whether the suture is continuous or interrupted. At all times, the surrounding tissue should be supported when removing sutures or staples, and the direction of removal should not put undue tension on the united wound (McGregor 1989).

Skin grafts

Types of skin grafts

A skin graft can be defined as (Grabb & Smith 1979):

> A segment of dermis and epidermis which has been completely separated from its blood supply and donor-site attachment before being transplanted to another area of the body.

Skin grafts can be of various thickness. They include both split-thickness and full-thickness skin grafts. If direct closure by suturing is not possible, these grafts are used to replace skin following burns, trauma, infection, and wide surgical excision (for example, excision of skin cancers) (Francis 1998; Mendez-Eastman 2001).

'If direct closure by suturing is not possible, these grafts are used to replace skin.'

Skin grafts

This portion of the text discusses the following aspects of skin grafts:
- types of skin grafts;
- split-thickness skin grafts;
- full-thickness skin grafts;
- applying a graft;
- care of a graft;
- 'taking' of skin grafts;
- care of a donor site; and
- care after healing.

Split-thickness skin grafts

A split-thickness skin graft (STSG) includes all of the epidermis and a portion of the dermis. Common donor sites include the thigh, the upper arm, and the buttock. Less common donor sites include the back, abdominal wall, forearm, and scalp (Francis 1998; McGregor 1989).

An STSG can be applied at the time of surgery, or it can be delayed until haemostasis has been achieved. The harvested skin can be wrapped in saline-moistened gauze, placed in a sterile plastic container, and stored at 4 degrees Celsius for up to 14–21 days (McGregor 1989).

Full-thickness skin grafts

A full-thickness graft (Wolfe graft) contains the epidermis and the entire thickness of the dermis (Grabb & Smith 1979). These grafts are usually small.

Donor skin can come from the post-auricular, pre-auricular, supra-clavicular, upper eyelid, antecubital, inguinal, hand, scalp, prepuce, labia majora, and areolar regions (Francis 1998). The skin-graft donor site is selected to match, as closely as possible, the area to be grafted.

'The skin-graft donor site is selected to match, as closely as possible, the area to be grafted.'

Donor sites are often directly closed with sutures. The graft itself is usually secured with sutures and a tie-over dressing (McGregor 1989).

Applying a graft

Before the graft is applied, the recipient bed should be free from infection and have a clean, well-vascularised (but not bleeding) wound bed.

To ensure that the graft 'takes', nursing management is aimed at supporting the revascularisation of the graft. For this to occur, the graft should (Francis 1998; McGregor 1989; Mendez-Eastman 2001):

- be immobilised to prevent friction and shear at the graft site;
- have close contact with the recipient bed (with fluid or clot not being allowed to accumulate under the graft);
- not be dependent (especially on the leg) because the hydrostatic pressure can 'lift' the graft; and
- be cared for using aseptic techniques to prevent wound infection.

Care of a graft

The graft should be cleansed to prevent exudate accumulating on, around, or under the graft. This might require aspiration or fenestration (nicking) of the graft to allow fluid to escape.

Friction and shear forces on the graft should be avoided at all times to avoid disruption to the immature and fragile vascularisation process (Mendez-Eastman, 2001).

Some skin grafts are left intact for 5–7 days with a pressure-type dressing. Emollient ointment can be used to protect and moisturise the graft.

'Taking' of skin grafts

The thicker the skin graft, the longer it takes to heal or 'take'. The process of graft 'take' includes a number of stages. These are (Francis 1998; Grabb & Smith 1979; Mendez-Eastman 2001):

- *fibrin adhesion*—initial adherence;
- *plasmatic imbibition*—plasma-like fluid absorbed from the graft;
- *inosculation of blood vessels*—vascular buds grow into the graft; and
- *establishment of lymphatic drainage*.

A graft that has 'taken' becomes pink and adheres to the underlying recipient bed.

Care of a donor site

Donor sites for split-thickness grafts are allowed to heal by secondary intention. They are often more painful than the grafted site. Dressings vary, but can include alginates, hydrocolloids, and retention sheets (Francis 1998; Mendez-Eastman 2001). These are often left in place for 10–14 days, but this varies according to the anatomical site, the person's age, and general healing capacity.

As noted above, donor sites for full-thickness grafts are often directly closed with sutures.

Care after healing

Both the graft and the donor site require additional care once they are healed. Particular attention should be paid to the following.

- Grafts on the lower limb might require supportive bandaging or stockings for up to six weeks.
- Graft and donor sites should be protected from sun damage by using protective clothing and sun-block agents.
- Graft and donor sites should be moisturised with non-perfumed moisturising agents.

Over time, the graft and donor site undergo texture and colour changes, and gradually fade.

Flaps

Definition and types

Flaps are a type of graft that involve tissue *with a network of blood vessels.*

Flaps can be classified in various ways. They can be classified according to their:

- *tissue composition*—for example: skin, fasciocutaneous, myocutaneous, osteomyocutaneous, or omental;
- *locality*—local or distant; or
- *vasculature*—for example: axial pattern, random pattern, free.

Depending on the classification used, flaps are described in various ways. The Box below contains some examples of this terminology.

Terminology used to describe flaps

Flaps can be classified according to their tissue, locality, or vasculature. This leads to various terms being used to describe flaps. These terms include the following.

Local and distant flaps

A *local flap* is in the immediate vicinity of the defect. Depending on the surgical technique that is used, they are sometimes described as a 'transposition', a 'rotation', or an 'advancement flap'. A *distant flap* is moved from one anatomical location to a distant wound site.

Free flaps and pedicle flaps

Free flaps have their blood supply separated from the original site. This is then re-established using microsurgical anastomosis of vessels at the recipient site. *Pedicle flaps* have their existing blood supply preserved as the flap is shifted to a new site.

Composite flaps

Composite flaps contain a combination of tissue types—for example, bone and skin (osteocutaneous) or muscle and skin (myocutaneous).

Indications

Flaps are used if:

- it is likely that a skin graft will not 'take'; or
- if durable tissue cover is required to protect underlying structures.

Flaps are of particular importance if bone, tendon, blood vessels, or nerves are exposed, or if it is necessary to reconstruct a defect with tissue of a similar quality—for example, in trans-rectus abdominis muscle (TRAM) flap breast reconstruction following mastectomy (Sandau 2002).

Pre-operative care

As with any patient with a wound, body image and changes in appearance and self-image are important issues. People who are undergoing reconstructive surgery therefore require education, counselling, and reassurance.

People who are to undergo flap surgery—whether minor or major—should be given a clear understanding of the procedure being planned, the post-operative care that will be needed, and the likely appearance of the flap. It is not uncommon for the flap to be oedematous post-operatively. However, patients should be reassured that this will subside, and that some flap shrinkage will occur over time. Larger flaps can create a secondary defect that requires skin grafting or delayed closure.

'As with any patient with a wound, body image and changes in appearance and self-image are important issues.'

Post-operative care

Nurses have a key role to play in the post-operative care of skin flaps. It is important to ensure (Clamon & Netscher 1994; Dinman & Giovannone 1994):

- adequate flap perfusion;
- temperature control;
- pain control; and
- monitoring for signs of infection.

Each of these is discussed below.

Flap perfusion

The person should be kept well hydrated. Oral and intravenous fluid intake should be closely monitored—along with pulse rate, blood pressure, and urine output. Blood pressure monitoring is vital. Both hypertension and hypotension are to be avoided.

'Blood pressure monitoring is vital. Both hypertension and hypotension are to be avoided.'

The flap should be carefully monitored for signs of arterial or venous compromise. This includes assessment of:

- the colour;
- temperature;
- tissue turgor; and
- capillary refill.

In some instances, Doppler assessment and dermal bleeding tests might be required.

In flaps in which kinking of the blood supply might occur (such as pedicle flaps), correct positioning is important to avoid compression or tension on the blood vessels (Dinman & Giovannone 1994; Maksud 1992).

'Correct positioning is important to avoid compression or tension on the blood vessels.'

Smoking is absolutely contraindicated, and caffeine intake might also have to be restricted. Both of these cause vasoconstriction.

Temperature control

The flap should be kept warm to prevent vasoconstriction. Thermal warming blankets and room-temperature regulation are key strategies to promote normothermia.

In addition, core body temperature is monitored, along with other vital signs. Many surgeons set parameters within which these should be maintained.

Pain control

In addition to the important comfort needs of the person undergoing flap surgery, pain and anxiety should be avoided because these can contribute to hypertension. Prevention and management of pain is therefore a priority.

Monitoring for infection

Nurses should monitor for signs of infection—both local and systemic. General post-surgical care should be undertaken to avoid complications—such as chest infections, pressure ulcers, and deep vein thrombosis.

Topical negative pressure therapy

Definition and uses

Topical negative pressure therapy (TNPT) is also known by its trade name of 'VAC®' ('vacuum-assisted closure').

TNPT is used to assist healing in a variety of wounds. It can be used on pressure ulcers, wound defects secondary to surgery, skin grafts, dehisced wounds, draining wounds, burns, and traumatic wounds (Argenta & Morykwas 1997; Banwell 1999; Deva et al. 2000).

Topical negative pressure therapy

This portion of the text discusses the following aspects of topical negative pressure therapy (TNPT):

- definition and uses;
- mechanism of action;
- indications;
- contraindications and precautions;
- application of TNPT; and
- developments in TNPT.

Mechanism of action

The primary mechanism of TNPT is local 'suction' applied to a wound. This is done by applying negative pressure through a porous foam dressing which is sealed locally with a film dressing and connected to a motorised pump via tubing.

The mechanisms of action are thought to include (Banwell & Teot 2003):

- enhanced dermal perfusion;
- stimulation of granulation tissue;
- reduced accumulation of interstitial fluid and oedema;
- decrease in bacterial colonisation;
- control of exudate; and
- wound contraction (or 'reverse tissue expansion').

Indications

The main indications for TNPT include:

- traumatic wounds including burns and limb trauma (including bony involvement);
- infected wounds;
- abdominal and sternal dehiscence;
- skin graft fixation;
- wound bed preparation (Banwell & Teot 2003);
- pressure ulcers (stages II, III, and IV); and
- diabetic and venous leg ulcers.

TNPT is often used if there is a cavity defect present or substantial tissue loss. In some instances, TNPT is used because the patient has contraindications to surgery—including medical risk, multiple wounds, difficult post-operative care, previous multiple surgery, or patient or family refusal (Deva et al. 2000).

Contraindications and precautions

In considering the suitability of this therapy, extreme care must be taken if the patient has any clotting abnormalities, fistulae, or open body cavities. Care should also be taken following resection of malignancies (Banwell & Teot 2003).

Application of TNPT

Before TNPT is applied, the wound should be debrided of non-viable tissue—such as slough or necrotic tissue. The person receiving therapy will be aware of a 'pulling' sensation. There might be some initial discomfort, but this usually abates. If pain is reported on commencement of therapy, the pressure should be reduced to a manageable level, and then slowly increased.

The pump can be programmed to provide continuous or intermittent therapy, and the pressure gradient can be adjusted. Clinical guidelines are available from the manufacturers for different wound types. However, it is usual for therapy to be applied continuously at 125 mm Hg initially, and then changed to intermittent (cyclical) therapy after 24 hours.

Small portable TNPT units are available. These offer greater mobility and independence to the person receiving therapy. However, units of larger capacity are required for large tissue defects with high volumes of exudate.

Dressing changes vary. They might be performed every 48 hours or twice a week—depending on the characteristics of the wound (Banwell & Teot 2003).

Indications to stop TNPT include (Banwell & Teot 2003):

- excessive pain;
- psychological intolerance;
- lack of healing after one to two weeks;
- frank pus draining from the wound; and
- excessive bleeding or haematoma.

Developments in TNPT

TNPT has offered a new strategy for dealing with wounds that are difficult to heal, and it provides an alternative to surgery in some cases. Further research is being conducted to establish which wounds respond best, and which pressure gradients are optimal.

'TNPT has offered a new strategy for dealing with wounds that are difficult to heal, and it provides an alternative to surgery in some cases.'

Alternative interfaces and foam dressings have also been explored to avoid unnecessary tissue trauma with an actively granulating wound. New techniques that allow TNPT to be used in the presence of a closed wound-irrigation system are also being explored.

Such new technologies offer exciting alternative options for management of recalcitrant wounds and for the care of people who are not suited to surgery.

Conclusion

There are many options available for the repair and reconstruction of wounds. Suturing can be used to repair lacerations and cuts, and skin grafts can be used to cover partial- and full-thickness defects of varying size. Flap surgery is available to provide durable tissue coverage over exposed structures, and larger defects can be filled with microvascular reconstruction and free flap. TNPT is a useful adjunct therapy in healing wounds or in preparing them for later skin closure, skin graft, or flap repair.

'At all times, nurses must be aware of the person who has the wound, and should offer a caring and holistic approach to management.'

In all of these treatment options, the primary goal is wound closure with an acceptable cosmetic and functional result. The role of the nurse is very important in achieving this objective. At all times, nurses must be aware of the *person* who has the wound, and should offer a caring and holistic approach to management.

Chapter 10

Leg Ulcers

Sue Templeton

Introduction

Leg ulcers are a significant burden on patients, their families, and healthcare systems. Approximately 15% of persons over the age of 80 years suffer from a leg ulcer (Hewitt et al. 2003). Leg ulcers have a high rate of recurrence and some people endure many years of non-healing leg ulcers (Scully 1999). For healthcare systems, the financial cost of managing venous leg ulcers can amount to hundreds of millions of dollars per annum (Hewitt et al. 2003).

> *'Leg ulcers are a significant burden on patients, their families, and healthcare systems.'*

This chapter first discusses the assessment and treatment of leg ulcers *in general terms*. For specific advice on the assessment and management of particular types of leg ulcers, see 'Venous leg ulcers' (this chapter, page 151) and 'Arterial leg ulcers' (this chapter, page 161).

Causes of leg ulcers

There are many causes of leg ulcers. These include (Carville 2001):

- circulatory insufficiency;
- lymphatic disorders;

- haematological disorders;
- metabolic disorders;
- tumours;
- infections;
- trauma; and
- allergic responses.

Leg ulcers can occur spontaneously or they can develop following trauma (which can be otherwise relatively trivial). Although trauma can be the initial cause of a lower limb wound, failure of the wound to heal is often the result of underlying health conditions (Carville 2001). Any lower limb wound that does not heal within six weeks is classified and treated as a leg ulcer (Scully 1999), even if the wound was initially an acute wound.

'The main cause of leg ulcers is circulatory insufficiency—of the venous system, the arterial system, or both.'

The main cause of leg ulcers is circulatory insufficiency (Scully 1999). This can be insufficiency of the venous system, the arterial system, or both (Cullum & Roe 1998). If venous and arterial insufficiency have been excluded as the cause of an ulcer, further investigations are necessary.

Referral to an appropriate medical specialist is required for any leg ulcer in which (Morison et al. 1997; RCN 1998):

- the aetiology is unclear;
- the clinical picture is unusual; or
- there is inadequate response to treatment in four weeks.

Any atypical, non-healing leg ulcer requires a biopsy to exclude malignancy (RCN 1998). The case study in the Box on page 149 describes the management of the leg ulcer shown in Figure 10.1 (page 149). The case study shows the importance of a biopsy in diagnosing an atypical non-healing wound.

'Any atypical, non-healing leg ulcer requires a biopsy to exclude malignancy.'

Biopsy in an atypical non-healing ulcer

Mr C was a 90-year-old man who had been referred by his general practitioner to a community nursing centre for treatment of a leg ulcer. The leg ulcer is shown in Figure 10.1, below.

The nurse noted that the ulcer was:

- rapidly increasing in size (including depth)
- comprised of sloughy and necrotic tissue;
- malodorous; and
- surrounded by rolled edges.

The nurse liaised with the general practitioner to arrange review of Mr C by a plastic surgeon. The plastic surgeon performed a biopsy which confirmed that the ulcer was a squamous cell carcinoma.

Surgery to excise the tumour was then performed.

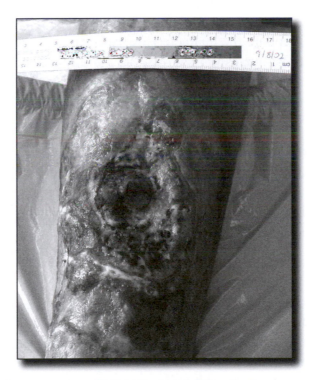

Figure 10.1 Squamous cell carcinoma of lower leg
Reproduced with permission of RDNS SA Inc.

Assessment

General principles of assessment

A comprehensive health history identifies factors that might impair wound healing in general and leg ulcers in particular. (For more on assessment of wounds in general, see Chapter 3, page 33.)

'It is important to assess the whole person, his or her limb, and the ulcer itself.'

To determine ulcer aetiology, nurses should undertake a comprehensive, systematic, documented assessment. It is important to assess the whole person, his or her limb, and the ulcer itself (Harker 2002).

Leg-ulcer assessment tools

A specialised tool for assessment of leg ulcers can be useful for identifying the characteristics that indicate various aetiologies—in particular, for differentiating between venous and arterial leg ulcers. Tools that utilise prompts to differentiate the characteristics specific to venous and arterial leg ulcers can assist nurses to reach a timely and accurate diagnosis. (For more on the introduction and use of such tools, see Chapter 3, 'Assessment and Documentation', page 33.)

Specific investigations

Specific investigations can be used to assist in establishing aetiology. Some of these are relatively simple and can be undertaken at the bedside or in the community. Other investigations need the facilities of a vascular laboratory or radiology department.

Multidisciplinary assessment

Assessment is often multidisciplinary and can involve input from the person, his or her general practitioner, nurses, medical specialists, radiologists, and allied health professionals. Timely and open communication among all members of the healthcare team promotes effective and efficient care—which optimises clinical outcomes.

Examination of the limb

Examination of the whole limb can reveal clues to assist in determining the aetiology of a leg ulcer. However, signs can vary, and the integration of a range of information obtained from all aspects of a comprehensive assessment is most likely to establish the aetiology of an ulcer.

Examination of the ulcer

Specific wound characteristics vary—depending on ulcer aetiology. Such factors as exudate level, wound dimensions, and tissue type in the ulcer base determine appropriate dressings and other management strategies. Wound progress is best monitored through regular systematic documentation (Harker 2002).

Treatment objectives

The general objectives of treatment of leg ulcers are (Carville 2001):

- identification and control (or elimination) of the underlying cause of the wound;
- improvement of circulation (if possible);
- promotion of optimal conditions for healing; and
- implementation of strategies (in conjunction with the person) to prevent recurrence and to maintain quality of life.

Once the aetiology of a leg ulcer has been determined, an individually planned management regimen should be developed. Because most leg ulcers are due to venous insufficiency or arterial insufficiency (or a combination of the two), the chapter will now consider each of these in more detail.

Venous leg ulcers

Venous systems in the lower limb

There are three systems of veins in the lower limbs—*deep veins*, *perforating veins*, and *superficial veins*. All veins contain valves. These reduce hydrostatic pressure when standing, and assist in returning blood to the heart.

The *deep veins* are the popliteal and tibial veins. These veins, which are located deep within the muscles of the leg, have few valves and a relatively high hydrostatic pressure.

The *superficial venous system* lies outside the fascia of the leg. It is comprised of the long and short saphenous veins. These veins have many valves and a low hydrostatic pressure.

The *perforators* (or communicating veins) connect the superficial and deep veins.

Pathophysiology of leg ulcers

Efficient venous return relies on a number of factors—especially effective muscular action in the lower legs and competent valves in the veins (see Table 10.1, below).

Table 10.1 Factors influencing efficient venous return
AUTHOR'S PRESENTATION (ADAPTED FROM MORISON ET AL. 1997; CULLUM & ROE 1998)

Factor	Relevance to venous return
Functioning of calf muscles (ability to plantar-flex and dorsi-flex ankle joint)	Contraction of calf muscles squeezes deep veins and pushes blood along veins
Functioning of valves in veins	Functional valves prevent backflow and pooling of blood in the venous system (venous hypertension)
Variations in intra-abdominal and intra-thoracic pressure	Pressure changes affect blood flow to and from the heart

Venous insufficiency of the deep veins accounts for the majority of leg ulcers (Cullum & Roe 1998). If the valves in the veins fail, increased pressure occurs within the deep venous system. This is transmitted to the superficial venous system, leading to increased pressure in that system (Morison et al. 1997). This increased pressure then leads to various pathophysiological changes and certain clinical presentations. These are shown in Figure 10.2 (page 153). The developing pathophysiological changes are shown on the left side of the diagram, and the various clinical manisfestations at each stage are shown on the right side of the diagram—culminating in venous ulcer formation.

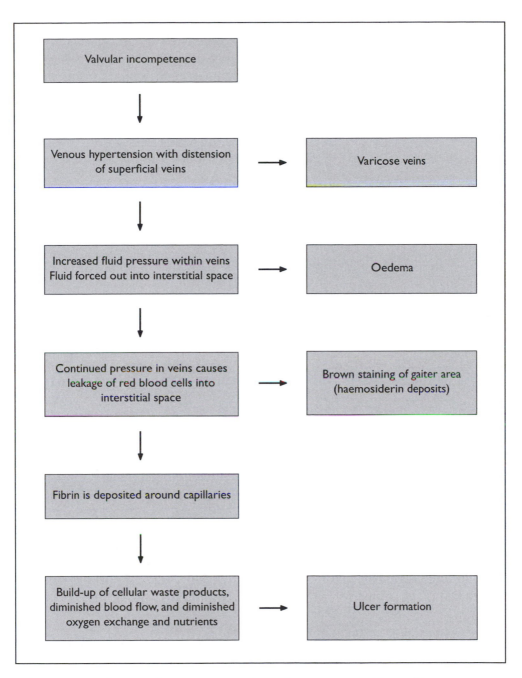

Figure 10.2 Pathophysiology and clinical presentation of venous insufficiency

AUTHOR'S PRESENTATION (ADAPTED FROM THOMAS 1998; HISLOP 1997); REPRODUCED WITH PERMISSION OF RDNS SA INC.

Conditions associated with venous insufficiency

Certain conditions are often associated with venous insufficiency. If nurses suspect that an ulcer is due to venous insufficiency, they should seek evidence of the following (Harker 2002; RCN 1998):

- a history of suspected or proven deep venous thrombosis, phlebitis, or pulmonary embolism;
- a history of surgery, fracture, or major trauma to the affected leg;
- varicose veins;
- obesity;
- immobility of lower limbs (such as muscle weakness, paraplegia); and
- restricted ankle joint movement.

Clinical appearance of venous ulcers

Ulcers that are due to venous insufficiency are likely to have certain typical features. Nurses should look for the signs and symptoms listed in the Box below.

Figure 10.3 (page 155) shows the typical appearance of a lower limb affected by venous insufficiency.

Signs and symptoms of a venous ulcer

The signs and symptoms of a venous ulcer include the following:

- an ulcer in the gaiter region of the leg (the lower one-third of the leg including the ankle);
- oedema of the lower limb (particularly after the limb has been in a dependent position);
- the presence of foot pulses—unlike arterial ulcers, venous ulcers are usually associated with normal foot pulses (although foot pulses can be difficult to palpate in the presence of oedema);
- a shallow ulcer with poorly defined margins;
- itchy, eczematous skin of the lower limb;
- red–brown pigmentation of gaiter area;
- slow ulcer progression;

(continued)

(continued)

- mild-to-moderate pain (usually not severe);
- relief of discomfort on elevation of the limb;
- red granulation tissue in the ulcer base;
- warm limb; and
- normal or rapid capillary return.

ADAPTED FROM CARVILLE (2001) AND VOWDEN, P. (1998)

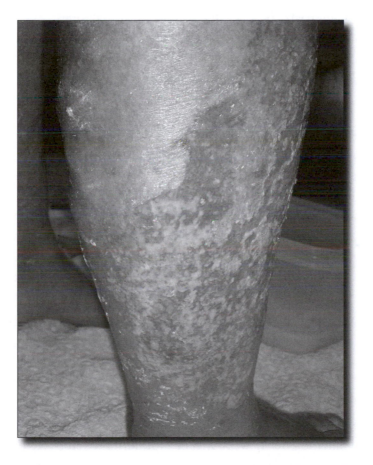

Figure 10.3 Typical appearance of a lower limb affected by venous insufficiency

Skin conditions associated with venous insufficiency

Certain skin conditions are commonly associated with venous insufficiency. These include:

- lipodermatosclerosis;
- atrophie blanche; and
- eczema.

  Each of these is discussed below.

Lipodermatosclerosis

Lipodermatosclerosis is a collection of skin changes associated with venous insufficiency. The condition results from chronic inflammation, fat necrosis, and scar tissue (Vowden, K. 1998). It usually occurs on the gaiter region of the leg. The condition presents with:

- red–brown skin pigmentation;
- oedema; and
- fibrosis of subcutaneous tissue.

  Although lipodermatosclerosis can present as an acute condition, it gradually worsens into a chronic state, and ulceration eventually occurs. The gaiter area can become very hard due to calcification of the subcutaneous tissues. Progression of lipodermatosclerosis can lead to the leg taking on the shape of an 'inverted champagne bottle'—when the gaiter area becomes fibrosed, while the calf above remains soft and oedematous (see Figure 10.4, page 157).

  Compression therapy is the appropriate treatment for lipodermatosclerosis. Although this treatment controls the condition, it is not curative.

Atrophie blanche

Atrophie blanche occurs when small areas of grey–white scar tissue form in areas of haemosiderin deposits or lipodermatosclerosis (Vowden, K. 1998). This is due to thrombosis and destruction of capillaries in the deep dermis, resulting in these areas becoming avascular.

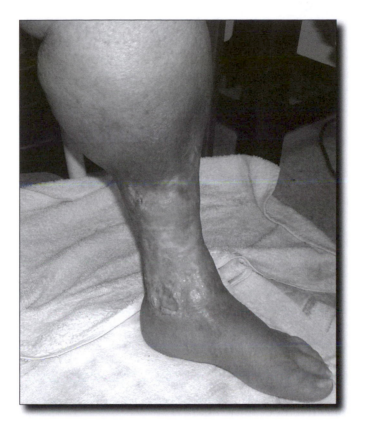

Figure 10.4 'Inverted champagne bottle' leg due to lipodermatosclerosis
REPRODUCED WITH PERMISSION OF RDNS SA INC.

Eczema

Eczema of the lower limb is a common occurrence in association with venous insufficiency. It presents as erythematous, scaly skin that can weep and is often itchy (Cullum & Roe 1998).

People with venous insufficiency also frequently demonstrate allergic or irritant contact dermatitis (Dowsett 2001). This can be caused by topical applications, dressings, and bandages (SIGN 1998). Patch testing of the person can assist nurses in choosing products that do not aggravate the condition.

Palpation of foot pulses

Palpation of foot pulses can provide guidance in differentiating between venous insufficiency and arterial insufficiency—although this is not definitive. Absent or weak foot pulses can indicate poor arterial blood supply. However, absent foot pulses can also be due to other causes (Vowden & Vowden 1996a). These include:

- oedema;
- congenital absence of the dorsalis pedis artery; and
- poor palpation technique.

Diagnosis should not therefore be based on the quality of foot pulses alone (see also 'Ankle–brachial pressure index', under 'Arterial leg ulcers', page 165).

Investigations

A number of investigations can be undertaken to confirm the presence of venous insufficiency. These include:

- ankle–brachial pressure index;
- duplex ultrasound;
- photoplesthysmography; and
- other investigations.

These are discussed below.

Ankle–brachial pressure index

Ankle–brachial pressure index (ABPI) is considered in greater detail below when arterial leg ulcers are discussed (see 'Ankle–brachial pressure index', under 'Arterial leg ulcers', page 165). However, in the context of venous ulcers, it should be noted that this index can be useful in both the *assessment* and *management* of venous ulcers.

With regard to *assessment*, ABPI can help to exclude arterial insufficiency as a cause of a leg ulcer—thus making the diagnosis of venous insufficiency more likely.

With regard to *management*, compression bandaging for venous ulcers is not recommended unless arterial insufficiency has been excluded by estimation of ABPI.

Duplex ultrasound

Duplex ultrasound is a specialised form of Doppler ultrasound (see page 165, this chapter, for more on Doppler). Duplex ultrasound uses continuous wave and pulsed Doppler.

Duplex ultrasound can produce (Iannos 1998):

- a visual display of tissue;
- the velocity of wave forms; and
- colour mapping of blood flow in real time.

Photoplesthysmography

Photoplesthysmography is a test used to determine the severity of venous valvular incompetence. Infrared light is emitted and reflected to assess venous refilling time following exercise (Vowden, P. 1998).

Other investigations

Other investigations that are performed in some centres include (Vowden, P. 1998):

- ambulatory venous pressure measurement;
- plethysmography;
- venography; and
- transcutaneous oxygen measurements.

Treatment of venous leg ulcers

Compression therapy

Graduated compression therapy is the foundation of venous leg ulcer treatment (Mear & Moffatt 2002). Compression therapy is covered in detail in Chapter 11 (page 171).

Adjunct measures

Adjunct measures to promote healing include (RCN 1998):

- leg elevation—this aids venous return and reduces swelling and pain; and
- exercise—moderate exercise using a heel–toe walking action maintains calf muscle pump function.

Dressings

Dressings alone are unlikely to heal a venous leg ulcer (SIGN 1998). In the early stages of treatment an absorbent wound dressing might be needed under compression therapy to absorb the large amounts of exudate. A dressing that is suitable for use under compression therapy should be chosen. If there is any doubt about the suitability of a dressing, the manufacturer's recommendations should be checked. Once the exudate is reduced, a simple, non-adherent dressing will suffice (RCN 1998).

'Dressings alone are unlikely to heal a venous leg ulcer.'

The limb and ulcer can be washed in tap water of drinking quality (SIGN 1998).

Venous eczema responds to topical corticosteroids (SIGN 1998). Other treatment options include zinc paste bandages and paraffin-based emollients. Lanolin, antiseptics, preservatives, and bandages containing latex should be avoided (SIGN 1998).

Surgery

Plastic surgery and venous surgery both have a role to play in the management of venous ulcers.

Plastic surgery using split skin grafts can accelerate the healing of venous leg ulcers, but this must be accompanied by the use of graded compression therapy (SIGN 1998).

Venous surgery can aid healing—particularly for superficial venous insufficiency in the presence of normal deep veins (SIGN 1998). Graded compression therapy should be worn following venous surgery.

A person's suitability for surgery is dependent on individual assessment by a medical specialist.

Long-term care of venous insufficiency

Once a venous leg ulcer has healed, the possibility of recurrence is high. Several strategies can be implemented to reduce the recurrence rate (Scully 1999; Nelson et al. 1996). These include the following.

- *Wearing below-knee compression stockings:* The stockings need to be fitted correctly, and replaced regularly and frequently. Refer to Chapter 11 (page 171) for further information.
- *Protecting healed skin:* This can be achieved through frequent use of moisturiser, avoiding trauma and constrictive garments, and frequent inspection of skin integrity.
- *Avoiding causative factors:* People should be advised to maintain acceptable weight, avoid crossing of legs, and elevate legs when sitting.
- *Prompt attention to skin breakdown:* People should be advised to seek professional assistance promptly if skin breakdown or injury occurs.
- *Assessing ankle–brachial pressure index (ABPI) every three months:* This will detect arterial disease early and allow for reassessment of treatment if necessary. (See page 165, this chapter, for notes on ABPI.)

Long-term care of venous ulcers

This section of the text discusses the long-term care of venous ulcers. In summary, the principles of long-term care are as follows:

- wearing below-knee compression stockings;
- protecting healed skin
- avoiding causative factors;
- prompt attention to skin breakdown; and
- assessing ankle–brachial pressure index (ABPI) every three months.

Arterial leg ulcers

Apart from venous insufficiency, the most common cause of leg ulcers is arterial insufficiency. Arterial leg ulcers result from a lack of arterial blood supply—leading to tissue ischaemia and necrosis. This is usually due to atherosclerosis and calcification of the arteries.

Atherosclerosis develops over time. However, it might not be clinically evident until the vessel has narrowed by 60%—producing ischaemia (Rice 1998).

As arterial disease worsens, collateral circulation and arteriolar dilatation develop in an effort to compensate and maintain adequate blood supply to the limb (Vowden & Vowden 1996b).

Conditions associated with arterial insufficiency

Certain conditions are associated with arterial insufficiency. If nurses suspect that an ulcer is due to arterial insufficiency, they should seek evidence of the following (Carville 2000; Rice 1998):

- diabetes mellitus;
- rheumatoid arthritis;
- a history of myocardial infarction, transient ischaemic attacks, or cerebrovascular accident;
- a history of angioplasty or arterial bypass surgery;
- ischaemic heart disease or other cardiac disease;
- hypertension;
- hyperlipidaemia; and
- cigarette smoking.

Clinical indications of arterial disease

The signs and symptoms of arterial disease vary—depending on the severity of vessel occlusion and the degree of compensatory effects.

The effects of ischaemia can produce:

- intermittent claudication; and
- critical ischaemia.

These are discussed below.

Intermittent claudication

Intermittent claudication is a common symptom of moderate arterial insufficiency. Intermittent claudication is characterised by cramping of the muscles distal to an arterial obstruction. It is brought on by exercise.

The pain results from insufficient arterial blood flow to meet the extra demands of exercise (Rice 1998).

Resting relieves the pain. As arterial insufficiency worsens, the amount of exercise required to produce symptoms is reduced and the rest time required to relieve symptoms increases.

Critical ischaemia

If arterial insufficiency becomes severe, blood flow at rest is inadequate to meet tissue demands. Critical ischaemia results. Signs and symptoms can be acute or chronic.

Chronic critical limb ischaemia is defined as (Vowden & Vowden 1996b):

- constant rest pain requiring regular analgesia for more than two weeks (with an ankle systolic blood pressure of less than 50 mm Hg); or
- ulceration or necrosis of the foot or toes (with the same blood pressure).

A line of demarcation can develop—with the distal limb appearing bright red when dependent, but pale on elevation.

'Complete arterial occlusion is a medical emergency.'

Complete arterial occlusion is a medical emergency. 'Complete arterial occlusion requires urgent treatment, such as endovascular thrombectomy or surgical exploration, to save the person's limb and life' (Rice 1998, p. 34). Unfortunately, critical limb ischaemia often results in amputation.

When an artery becomes occluded the clinical signs are referred to as 'the five Ps'. These are:

- pain;
- pallor;
- pulselessness;
- paraesthesia; and
- paralysis.

Clinical appearance of arterial ulcers

Ulcers that are due to arterial insufficiency are likely to have certain typical features. Nurses should look for the signs and symptoms listed in the Box below. Figure 10.5 (page 165) shows the typical appearance of an arterial ulcer.

Signs and symptoms of an arterial ulcer

Clinical signs and symptoms of arterial ulcers include:

- an absence of oedema;
- an ulcer on the malleolus, foot, or toes (but can also appear on the gaiter area);
- weak or absent pulses;
- cool limb with slow capillary return;
- deep ulcer with a 'punched-out' appearance;
- rapid progression;
- severe pain that can require narcotic analgesia for relief;
- pain reported as worse at night or on limb elevation;
- an ulcer base often containing sloughy and/or necrotic tissue; and
- thickened toenails, absence of leg and foot hair, and shiny skin.

ADAPTED FROM CARVILLE (2001) AND DEALEY (1994)

This chapter has now presented the typical signs and symptoms of a venous ulcer (Box, page 154) and the typical signs and symptoms of an arterial ulcer (Box, above). For convenience, these are summarised in a comparison table (Table 10.2, page 153). However, it should be noted that this table is for guidance only. A definitive diagnosis requires an overall assessment, including special investigations and specialist referral as appropriate.

Investigations

The most common investigations to determine the severity of arterial disease are ankle–brachial pressure index (ABPI) and angiography. These are discussed below.

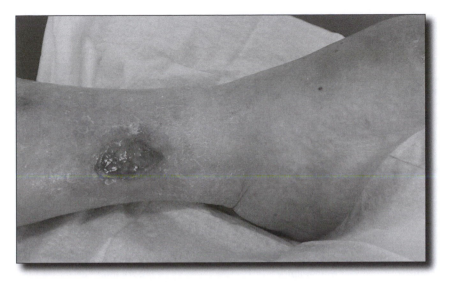

Figure 10.5 Typical appearance of an arterial ulcer
REPRODUCED WITH PERMISSION OF RDNS SA INC.

Other investigations that might be available in some centres include measurement of segmental limb pressures, magnetic resonance imaging (MRI), diagnostic angioscopy, intravascular ultrasound, and angiography with carbon dioxide (Morris & Kerstein 2001).

Ankle–brachial pressure index

The ankle–brachial pressure index (ABPI) is calculated using Doppler ultrasound to assist in determining the presence and severity of arterial disease. However, the ABPI is only one component of a comprehensive assessment of leg ulcers. It should be used as an adjunct to the clinical picture, but should not replace a comprehensive clinical assessment.

The ABPI is a ratio that compares the peak arm systolic blood pressure with peak ankle systolic blood pressure (Vowden & Vowden 2001). The ratio is ascertained by Doppler ultrasound using a simple, non-invasive technique that can be undertaken in a hospital, clinic, or home. The Doppler technique uses 'high-frequency scanning sound to detect the velocity and flow of blood in arteries and veins' (Anderson 1995, p. 325). Differences in arterial blood flow result in differences in audible sound frequency as detected by Doppler ultrasound (Iannos 1998).

Table 10.2 Comparison of signs and symptoms of venous and arterial ulcers

AUTHOR'S PRESENTATION (ADAPTED FROM CARVILLE 2001; DEALEY 1994; VOWDEN, P. 1998)

Characteristic	Venous ulcers	Arterial ulcers
Location	gaiter region of the leg (lower one-third of the leg including the ankles)	malleolus, foot, or toes (but can also appear on the gaiter area)
Oedema	oedema of the lower limb (particularly after the limb has been in a dependent position)	absent
Pulses	usually present—although foot pulses can be difficult to palpate in the presence of oedema	weak or absent pulses
Temperature	warm limb	cool limb
Capillary return	normal or rapid capillary return	slow capillary return
Appearance	shallow ulcer with poorly defined margins; red granulation tissue in ulcer base	deep ulcer with a 'punched-out' appearance; ulcer base often containing sloughy and/or necrotic tissue
Progression	slow	rapid
Pain	mild-to-moderate pain (usually not severe); relief of discomfort on elevation of the limb	severe pain that can require narcotic analgesia for relief; pain reported as worse at night or on limb elevation
Associated skin changes	itchy, eczematous skin of the lower limb; red–brown pigmentation of gaiter area	thickened toenails; absence of leg and foot hair; shiny skin

The ABPI assists in determining the presence and severity of arterial disease. It is used as an adjunct to a comprehensive clinical assessment, and provides valuable information that might not be obtained by clinical examination alone (Anderson 1995).

Although there is a common misunderstanding that a normal ABPI confirms venous insufficiency, it is important to note that ABPI neither confirms nor excludes venous insufficiency. A normal ABPI can indicate that an ulcer is less likely to be due to arterial insufficiency, but it does not prove that the ulcer is necessarily due to venous insufficiency.

The clinical relevance of ABPI results is outlined in Table 10.3 (below).

Table 10.3 ABPI values and interpretation
AUTHOR'S PRESENTATION

ABPI value	Interpretation
Greater than 1.30	Incompressible vessels; results not useful
1.01–1.30	Possible partial incompressibility; correlate with clinical assessment
0.90–1.00	Normal peripheral arterial circulation
0.80–0.90	Slight deficit in peripheral arterial circulation; correlate with clinical assessment
0.50–0.85	Arterial impairment might exist; referral to vascular specialist recommended
Less than 0.50	Significantly reduced arterial circulation; urgent referral to vascular specialist required

Caution must be exercised when interpreting ABPI results in certain circumstances. These include the following.

- People with diabetes can have arterial calcification, and this can result in falsely high ABPI results (Vowden & Vowden 1996a). To overcome this, measurement of toe systolic blood pressure is recommended (Morris & Kerstein 2001).
- Repeatedly inflating the sphygmomanometer cuff (or prolonged cuff inflation) can cause a hyperaemic response resulting in a falsely low ankle-pressure reading.
- An irregular heart beat (such as in atrial fibrillation) can make it difficult to obtain the systolic blood pressure (Vowden & Vowden 1996a).

To ensure that nurses are competent to perform the procedure and interpret the findings, they should undertake an educational program that includes: (i) an understanding of how Doppler ultrasound works; (ii) the procedure for obtaining ABPI; (iii) interpretation of the results; and (iv) limitations and precautions (Hislop 1997).

Angiography

Angiography involves the injection of radio-opaque dye into an artery. X-rays are then taken as the dye flows through the vessels.

Angiography provides detailed information on the location and severity of arterial blockage. However, it is an invasive procedure with several risks.

Treatment of arterial leg ulcers

Specialist consultation

Arterial ulceration is best managed in conjunction with a vascular surgeon. A vascular surgeon can assess arterial disease severity, determine a definitive diagnosis, and discuss treatment options with the person (Carville 2001).

'Arterial ulceration is best managed in conjunction with a vascular surgeon.'

Nursing objectives

Nursing objectives include the control of risk factors (if possible), prevention of infection, and sound wound-management practices (Morison et al. 1997). Regular exercise can help to develop collateral circulation—which leads to a decrease in symptoms (Rice 1998).

Compression bandaging

Compression bandaging is not used with persons who have arterial disease. This restricts circulation that is already compromised and can cause severe tissue damage (Cullum & Roe 1998).

Dressings

Ulcers due to severe arterial disease are very unlikely to heal with dressings alone (Smith 2002). Dressings should be chosen according to the needs of the person, the wound characteristics, and long-term objectives.

Because of the reduced blood supply, infection is a major risk. Dressings such as cadexomer iodine and silver dressings are therefore useful for their antimicrobial properties.

Occlusive adhesive dressings should be avoided because these can damage fragile skin. Arterial ulcers can be present for many years, and a dressing that provides a moist wound environment is therefore recommended. The chosen dressings should be comfortable and acceptable to the person, as well as being simple and cost-effective. The variety and combination of ulcer treatments should be kept to a minimum (Cullum & Roe 1998).

Surgery

Surgical options for the treatment of arterial ulcers aim to improve the arterial supply. A person's suitability for surgery is dependent on health status, other conditions, and the nature and extent of arterial disease.

Possible interventions include (Carville 2001; Morris & Kerstein 2001):

- chemical or surgical sympathectomy;
- angioplasty (balloon or stent);
- atherectomy;
- vascular bypass surgery; and
- amputation.

Mixed vessel ulcers

Some ulcers can be due to a combination of venous and arterial disease. A thorough assessment and an individualised treatment plan are required to manage this challenging problem.

Treatment options and patient outcomes are dependent on the degree of arterial disease and patient factors (such as suitability for surgery). Referral to a vascular specialist for expert assessment is recommended.

Light compression bandaging can be used if the degree of arterial disease is not severe (Smith 2002).

Other aetiologies

Diabetes mellitus can cause arterial disease, venous disease, and neuropathy (autonomic, sensory, and motor neuropathy). All of these conditions can contribute to lower limb ulcers. Management of people with diabetes is discussed in Chapter 14 (page 229).

Other pathologies can be responsible for leg ulcers. A discussion of the effects of trauma can be found in Chapter 8 (page 121), and a discussion of dermatological conditions can be found in Chapter 18 (page 299).

Conclusion

Nurses play a vital role in the management of leg ulcers. Armed with a sound knowledge and skill base, nurses can assess, plan, and implement a management regimen and evaluate the person's response. Nurses are also often in a position to coordinate the multidisciplinary team.

'A leg ulcer is not a diagnosis. The identification of a leg ulcer is only the start of a collaborative relationship that aims to optimise outcomes for the person concerned.'

Nurses provide support and education to people living with leg ulcers. A leg ulcer is not a diagnosis. The identification of a leg ulcer is only the start of a collaborative relationship among the nurse, the person, and other health professionals—a relationship that aims to optimise outcomes for the person concerned.

Chapter 11

Bandaging and Compression Therapy

Sue Templeton

Introduction

Approximately 1–2% of people develop a chronic lower leg ulcer (Stacey et al. 2002). Although chronic lower leg ulceration occurs most commonly in older adults, it also affects a small proportion of younger adults (Hewitt et al. 2003). Approximately 55–70% of leg ulcers are due to venous hypertension (Hewitt et al. 2003; Rice 2002).

The aims of treatment of venous leg ulcers are: (i) to promote the return of fluid from the tissues into the vascular and lymphatic systems; and (ii) to facilitate venous return through support of the veins (Hofman 1998). This is achieved through the application of graded compression therapy to the affected limb.

Factors influencing venous return

Effective venous return from the lower limbs depends on pressure exerted by the calf muscles during exercise. This so-called 'calf-muscle pump' is the most important factor in promoting venous return (Vowden & Vowden 1998), and efficient venous return is impaired in people with limited capacity to walk or exercise (Rice 2002). To maximise the action of the calf-muscle pump, a functioning ankle joint and a 'heel–toe' walking action are necessary. Patent valves in the veins then prevent backflow of blood (Vowden & Vowden 1998). (For more on valves, see 'Venous systems in the lower limb', Chapter 10, page 151.)

Several conditions predispose to venous insufficiency. Limb immobility, pregnancy, long periods of standing, and severe heart failure can result in prolonged venous hypertension—thus leading to venous insufficiency (Vowden & Vowden 1998). Deep vein thrombosis, pulmonary embolus, venous surgery, or fracture of a leg can damage the veins and/or valves—thus producing venous insufficiency (Harker 2002). (For more on venous leg ulcer pathophysiology, see 'Pathophysiology of leg ulcers', Chapter 10, page 152.)

'Compression therapy controls venous insufficiency, but does not cure the condition.'

Graded compression therapy controls venous insufficiency, but does not cure the condition. Compression therapy is therefore necessary for as long as venous insufficiency exists. For most people, therapy must be continued all their lives (Nelson 1996).

Indications and contraindications

Indications for compression therapy

In the absence of clinically significant arterial disease, graded compression therapy is recognised as the definitive treatment for venous leg ulcers (Fletcher, Cullum & Sheldon 1997; Stacey 2002). Compression enhances the action of the calf-muscle pump and forces fluid from the tissues back into the vascular and lymphatic systems (Thomas 1996).

'In the absence of clinically significant arterial disease, compression therapy is recognised as the definitive treatment for venous leg ulcers.'

When correctly applied, compression garments provide a rigid casing around the leg. This overcomes the effects of high hydrostatic pressure within the veins (Thomas & Nelson 1998a). Hydrostatic pressure is greatest at the ankle

Framework of the chapter.

This chapter discusses bandaging and compression therapy under the following headings:

and decreases up the limb. The greatest level of compression is therefore required at the ankle (Thomas 1996).

Contraindications for compression therapy

If arterial blood flow is poor, compression therapy can reduce existing arterial perfusion to dangerously low levels (Stacey et al. 2002). Significant arterial disease must therefore be excluded before compression therapy is started. This requires a comprehensive assessment of the person with a leg ulcer. (For more on this, see 'Arterial ulcers', Chapter 10, page 161.)

'Significant arterial disease must be excluded before compression therapy is started.'

The science of compression therapy

Optimal pressures

A compression pressure of 30–40 mm Hg at the ankle is optimal for treatment of venous leg ulcers, grading to 15–20 mm Hg at the top of the calf (Thomas & Nelson 1998b; Rice 2002).

Continuous application of optimal compression pressure can heal 40–80% of venous leg ulcers in 12 weeks (Nelson 1996). Compression pressure of less than 15 mm Hg at the ankle is insufficient to provide any enhancement of venous return (Negus 1991). For people with existing oedema or large limbs, a compression pressure of greater than 20 mm Hg at the ankle is required (Thomas & Nelson 1998b).

Laplace's law

Compression pressure (also known as sub-bandage pressure) is governed by Laplace's law. According to Laplace's law:

$$P = (N \times T) / (C \times W)$$

where:

P = sub-bandage pressure

N = number of layers applied

T = bandage tension

C = limb circumference

W = bandage width

Laplace's law means that compression pressure is *directly proportional* to: (i) the tension of the bandage during application and (ii) the number of layers applied. Conversely, compression pressure is *inversely proportional* to: (i) the circumference of the limb and (ii) the width of the bandage.

In practical terms, Laplace's law means that compression pressure increases (Mear & Moffatt 2002):

- as the bandage tension (stretch) *increases*;
- as the number of bandage layers *increases*;
- as the limb circumference *decreases*; and
- as the bandage width *decreases* (that is, if a narrower bandage is used).

This means that when a bandage is applied using constant tension to a limb with a gradually increasing diameter (from the ankle to the top of the calf), graded compression will result (Thomas & Nelson 1998a).

Applying compression

Training

The skill level of the nurse significantly affects the level of compression achieved (Stockport et al. 1997). Incorrectly applied compression can result in inadequate or excessive compression pressure (RCN Institute 1998). Poor application technique can also result in increased ulcer size, pressure ulcers, ridging of the skin, blisters, and pain.

A training program with formal accreditation of the nurse's competency in application of compression bandages ensures skill and proficiency.

Technique for applying compression therapy

Nurses are advised to check individual manufacturer's recommendations regarding application of compression-bandage systems. The compression level and indications for use should be checked before applying any bandages, stockings, or pantyhose for the purpose of enhancing venous return.

'The compression system should completely cover the person's lower leg—from the base of the toes to the top of the calf.'

If possible, compression should be applied early in the day (when oedema is less). Caution should be exercised when commencing compression therapy for people with cardiac failure. Compression therapy causes a fluid shift from the leg tissues into the circulation, and this can exacerbate cardiac failure (Hampton 1998).

The person's foot should be positioned at 90 degrees to the lower leg during application of compression bandages (Hampton 1998). This prevents 'bunching' of the bandages at the top of the foot during dorsiflexion (which can result in tissue damage). The compression system should completely cover the person's lower leg—from the base of the toes to the top of the calf. The heel and sole of the foot must be included.

Unless otherwise stated for particular compression systems, compression-bandage systems are applied using the standard technique described in the Box on page 176.

Standard technique

The standard technique for applying a compression bandage is as follows:

- *Step 1:* Using a 'figure-of-eight' technique, the bandage is anchored on the foot and the heel is covered.
- *Step 2:* A spiral technique (with 50% bandage stretch and 50% overlap of the previous layer) is then used up the leg.
- *Step 3:* The bandage is finished at the top of the calf (approximately two finger-widths below the knee) (Hampton 1998).

Excess bandage should be cut off if it is too long. Winding a bandage around a limb multiple times at calf level (or bandaging back down the limb) can produce a tourniquet effect. More than one bandage should be used if necessary for large or long limbs. Inadequate overlap reduces the compression pressure.

'A correctly applied compression bandage system feels firm for the person, but not tight or constrictive.'

A correctly applied compression bandage system is not loose or puckered. It feels firm for the person, but not tight or constrictive.

Nurses should follow the manufacturer's recommendations regarding application, re-use, and washing of bandages and stockings.

A tubular retention bandage or stockingette can be useful over compression bandages to keep them in place and to prevent 'roll-up' overnight (Hampton 1998).

Reduced compression

A reduced level of compression can be used in certain instances. However, to enhance venous return, sustained compression pressure of at least 15 mm Hg at the ankle is necessary.

A reduced compression pressure can be considered:

- when first commencing compression (to enhance patient acceptance);
- if there is a mild degree of arterial insufficiency (Morison & Moffatt 1994); and
- if the person is resistant to, or cannot tolerate, a greater level of compression—despite education and support.

The most common method for achieving a reduced compression is to apply only three layers of a four-layer compression-bandage system (see 'Four-layer bandage systems', this chapter, page 180). Padding and crêpe bandage are applied in the usual manner. The nurse then applies a light elastic bandage or a cohesive bandage.

If optimal compression pressures cannot be achieved and maintained, ulcers can take longer to heal. People who have leg discomfort without significant arterial disease often find that their tolerance for compression increases as oedema reduces.

Dressings

Dressings are usually required over any ulcerated area to manage exudate and to provide a moist wound environment. Nurses should choose a dressing that is suitable for use under compression—such as one that 'locks' exudate within the dressing.

'Dressings are usually required over any ulcerated area to manage exudate and to provide a moist wound environment.'

Initially, an absorbent dressing is usually required due to high exudate levels. However, because compression reduces the oedema, the level of wound exudate usually decreases with time, and the suitability of the chosen dressing should therefore be reassessed at intervals.

Once the exudate has reduced, a simple, non-adherent dressing will suffice (RCN 1998). The limb and ulcer can be washed in tap water of drinking quality (SIGN 1998).

Padding

Padding is required under most compression-bandage systems. Padding:

- protects bony prominences;
- spreads bandage tension more evenly;
- provides some insulation; and
- aids comfort.

Padding should not be applied directly over an ulcer because it can adhere to the wound. A suitable dressing should be chosen.

'Padding should not be applied directly over an ulcer because it can adhere to the wound.'

Padding is available as a bandage or tubular sock. Bandage-type padding is applied using the standard technique (see Box, page 176). However, the bandage should be stretched only enough to prevent 'puckers'. If necessary, padding can be used to re-shape legs into the optimal conical shape to ensure graded compression (see Figure 11.1, below).

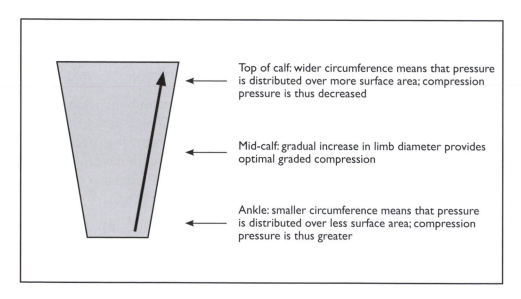

Top of calf: wider circumference means that pressure is distributed over more surface area; compression pressure is thus decreased

Mid-calf: gradual increase in limb diameter provides optimal graded compression

Ankle: smaller circumference means that pressure is distributed over less surface area; compression pressure is thus greater

Figure 11.1 Optimal limb shape for graded compression therapy
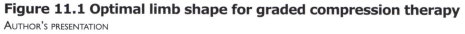
AUTHOR'S PRESENTATION

Extra padding might be required for people with slender calves, or legs with a narrow gaiter area—so-called 'inverted champagne bottle leg' (see Chapter 10, page 156). It is important to use extra padding for ankles of less than 18-cm circumference to prevent excessive compression pressure (Mear & Moffatt 2002).

'Inadequate padding can result in local tissue damage, including necrosis.'

Extra padding is often required over bony prominences—such as the tibial plateau (below the knee) and malleoli (ankles). The area over the Achilles tendon might also require extra padding. Inadequate padding can result in local tissue damage, including necrosis (Mear & Moffatt 1998).

Various types of padding are available. They can be composed of synthetic, natural, or blended fibres. Several companies produce foam products specifically designed for people with a prominent malleolus. These fill the space behind the malleolus to ensure that compression pressure is applied evenly (Rice 2002).

Types of compression systems

Choosing a compression-therapy system

There are several compression-therapy systems available for treatment of venous leg ulcers. These include:

- multi-layer bandages;
- short-stretch (inelastic) bandages;
- long-stretch (elastic) bandages; and
- hosiery.

Although it has been said that there ' ... is no basis for advocating any one particular high compression system' (Cullum et al. 1998, p. 2), there is some evidence that multi-layer

'There is some evidence that multi-layer bandage systems are more effective than single-layer systems.'

bandage systems are more effective than single-layer systems (Nelson & Thomas 1998).

The choice of a compression bandage system is made after giving consideration to patient factors, availability, cost, ability to re-use, ease of application, and the skills of the user. Table 11.1 (below) provides useful information in making a decision.

Table 11.1 Choosing a compression-bandage system
AUTHOR'S PRESENTATION

Issue	Comments
Mild arterial insufficiency	A short-stretch bandage is better tolerated by patients with mild arterial insufficiency
Cost-effectiveness	Long-stretch bandages and non-adhesive short-stretch bandages can be washed numerous times
Complaints of pain or discomfort	A short-stretch bandage is more comfortable at night (due to low resting pressure) Patients report that four-layer compression-bandage systems are comfortable
Ease of use	Short-stretch bandages are relatively easy to apply
Effectiveness	Compression of 30–40 mm Hg at the ankle is optimal for healing of venous leg ulcers; however, some compression is better than no compression
Patient factors	A four-layer compression bandage system is more difficult for the patient to remove or alter (due to the outer cohesive bandage) A short-stretch or long-stretch compression-bandage system can allow the patient to wear usual footwear
Allergy or sensitivity	Non-adhesive short-stretch bandages are 100% cotton In some countries, 'latex-free' four-layer compression-bandage systems are available

Four-layer bandage systems

Four-layer systems use four layers of bandage—(i) padding; (ii) crêpe bandage; (iii) light elastic bandage; and (iv) cohesive bandage. Only the third and fourth layers apply compression—17 mm Hg at the third layer and 23 mm Hg at the fourth layer (Smith & Nephew 2002). Correctly applied, a four-layer compression-bandage system maintains pressure of 40 mm Hg at the ankle for one week (Fletcher, Cullum & Sheldon 1997).

A four-layer compression-bandage system is applied in the manner described in the Box below.

Applying a four-layer compression system

The technique for applying a four-layer compression-bandage system is as follows:

- *Layer 1:* Padding—for application, see 'Padding', this chapter, page 178.
- *Layer 2:* Crêpe bandage—the crêpe bandage provides a smooth surface to which the light elastic bandage can conform; the crêpe bandage should be applied using standard technique.
- *Layer 3:* Light elastic bandage—using a 'figure-of-eight' technique, the bandage is anchored on the foot, and the heel is covered; a 'figure-of-eight' technique (with 50% stretch and 50% overlap) of the previous layer is then used up the leg.
- *Layer 4:* Cohesive bandage—applied using standard technique.

Patients are often unable to wear their usual footwear due to the bulk of the bandage. If the foot is pushed into person's usual shoes, the bandages can be pushed up. This reduces compression efficacy, and tissue damage can occur. A post-operative shoe or a large sturdy slipper can be worn during the treatment period to overcome this problem.

Some four-layer compression-bandage systems contain latex. Patients and nurses who are allergic to latex should therefore exercise caution.

Short-stretch bandages

This system uses an inelastic bandage (with less than 50% stretchability) applied over padding. Most of these short-stretch bandages are made of 100% cotton, although some have a light adhesive on one side to help prevent slipping.

Short-stretch bandages provide reduced pressure when the person is resting, and greater pressure when the person is exercising (Mear &

Moffatt 2002). Short-stretch bandages apply 25–35 mm Hg at the ankle when the patient is walking (Carville 2001). Walking enhances venous return as the calf muscles are compressed against the bandage.

Due to the inelasticity of the bandage, frequent reapplication might be necessary in the early stages as oedema is reduced (Thomas & Nelson 1998b). Once oedema has resolved, the bandage can be left in place for seven days.

'Due to the inelasticity of the bandage, frequent reapplication might be necessary in the early stages as oedema is reduced.'

The short-stretch bandage is applied using the standard technique with 90% stretch.

Long-stretch bandages

This system uses an elastic bandage (with greater than 50% stretchability) applied over padding. Some types of long-stretch bandages contain latex.

Long-stretch bandages provide high compression pressure at rest and during exercise. Although they do not need to be removed overnight, some people find that these bandages are uncomfortable at night because of the high resting pressure.

Many have shapes printed on them—which alter when the bandage is stretched. These assist nurses to achieve correct compression pressure.

The bandage should be applied using standard technique (Box, page 176). A correctly applied long-stretch compression bandage provides 40 mm Hg on an ankle of 18–25 cm circumference (Mear & Moffatt 2002; Cullum & Roe 1998).

Zinc-paste bandages

Although zinc-paste bandages do not provide compression, they can be very effective in treating lower-limb eczema associated with venous disease (Morison & Moffatt 1994). They can be applied directly over the ulcer, with a compression bandage over them.

There are several different types of zinc-paste bandages available. Some have additives—such as calamine, ichthammol, and coal tar. Because some zinc-paste bandages can constrict in certain conditions, they are

Compression systems and other therapies

This section of the text discusses the following compression systems and other therapies:

- four-layer bandages (page 180);
- short-stretch (inelastic) bandages (page 181);
- long-stretch (elastic) bandages (page 182);
- zinc paste bandages (page 182);
- retention bandages (page 183);
- Unna's boot (page 183);
- intermittent pneumatic-compression therapy (page 184);
- compression hosiery (page 184); and
- tubular bandages (page 186).

applied using a method of 'folding back' the bandage (Morison & Moffatt 1994). It is important to check the manufacturer's recommendations for application.

Zinc-paste bandages can remain in place for seven days.

Retention bandages

Retention bandages (such as crêpe bandages) do not provide enough compression to enhance venous return. Retention bandages can cause significant trauma if applied incorrectly or too tightly.

Other therapies

Unna's boot

Unna's boot is a rigid plaster-type dressing. In composition it is similar to a paste bandage, with the addition of glycerine. The bandage hardens— providing compression and a wound dressing (Cullum & Roe 1998).

There is no evidence that this therapy produces better healing rates than other compression systems (Cullum et al. 1998).

Intermittent pneumatic-compression therapy

Intermittent pneumatic-compression consists of a sleeve that encases the leg. This sleeve is attached to a pump. Cells in the sleeve inflate and deflate cyclically—according to a pre-determined sequence and pressure. This provides a 'milking effect' to enhance venous return.

Intermittent pneumatic-compression therapy normally delivers pressures of 30–50 mm Hg. Therapy is used at least twice a day for at least an hour each time (Carville 2001).

Intermittent pneumatic compression can improve healing rates of venous leg ulcers when used in association with compression stockings (see below) or Unna's boot (NHS 1997).

The major disadvantage is that the patient is unable to ambulate during therapy. In addition, this therapy requires a person skilled in application and removal of the device.

Compression hosiery

Graded compression hosiery is available in a range of compression levels, styles, and colours. Such stockings are usually worn once a venous leg ulcer has healed (Jones 1998).

As previously noted (page 172), compression controls venous insufficiency, but does not cure it. To prevent recurrence of venous insufficiency and possible re-ulceration, it is therefore necessary for people to wear such hosiery for the rest of their lives (Jones 1998).

'It is necessary for people to wear compression hosiery for the rest of their lives.'

It is best to choose stockings according to the pressure required at the ankle. Stockings are often classified into 'classes'. However, the range of pressures within different classes varies among countries. Nurses should check with each manufacturer to ensure that the correct stocking is chosen for the person. Table 11.2 (page 185) provides guidelines for stocking selection.

Stockings are usually removed immediately before bed and are reapplied as soon as possible after getting out of bed. However, some people leave their stockings on for two or three days at a time.

Table 11.2 Choosing a compression stocking

AUTHOR'S PRESENTATION

Compression (at ankle)	Description	Indications
15–20 mm Hg	Light support	Mild varicose veins
20–30 mm Hg	Medium support	Moderately severe varicose veins Prevention of venous leg ulcers Treatment of mild oedema
30–40 mm Hg	Strong support	Chronic venous insufficiency Severe varicose veins Treatment and prevention of venous leg ulcers
More than 50 mm Hg	Very strong support	Lymphoedema

Stockings of moderate-to-high compression can be difficult to apply and remove. A range of donning aids is available to assist. Wearing dishwashing gloves while putting stockings on provides good grip.

Stockings need to be replaced at least every six months, or when they have lost their elastic support due to wear or washing (Carville 2001). Reassessment before new stockings are purchased ensures that the correct compression pressure is achieved, and allows early detection of any arterial sufficiency.

'Reassessment before new stockings are purchased ensures that the correct compression pressure is achieved, and allows early detection of any arterial sufficiency.'

It is important to note that many brands of 'supermarket' pantyhose that purport to be useful for 'tired, aching legs' do not provide adequate compression to enhance venous return.

Anti-embolic stockings are indicated for prevention of deep vein thrombosis while legs are elevated in bed. Anti-embolic stockings do not provide adequate, sustained compression therapy while ambulating.

Tubular bandages

Tubular bandages are often used as an alternative to compression bandages or hosiery. They are available in parallel and shaped styles.

Parallel tubular bandages are unlikely to provide compression pressures above 15 mm Hg at the ankle, even when a double layer is applied. These bandages can produce a reverse pressure gradient due to their looseness at the ankle (Cullum & Roe 1998).

'Tubular bandages are not a substitute for a good compression bandaging.'

Shaped tubular bandages can provide some compression. However, this compression is unlikely to be clinically adequate for moderate-to-severe venous insufficiency.

Tubular bandages are not a substitute for a good compression bandaging (Cullum & Roe 1998).

Patient education

Education promotes compliance and empowerment of the person (Nelson 1996). For compression to be effective it must be worn continuously. Informing and supporting the person assists him or her to accept compression therapy.

The basic physiology of venous disease, the benefits of compression therapy, and how compression therapy will assist with ulcer healing should all be explained to the person. He or she should be informed that dressings alone are unlikely to heal venous leg ulcers and that compression therapy is the recognised path to healing.

'Dressings alone are unlikely to heal venous leg ulcers ... compression therapy is the recognised path to healing.'

The person should be encouraged to exercise because this facilitates the action of the calf-muscle pump and enhances venous return. Specific exercises to maintain maximum flexion of the ankle joint can be useful. When resting, elevation of the lower limbs reduces venous hydrostatic pressure.

Verbal and written information with reinforcement should be provided as required (Jones 1998). The person should be shown how to care for his or her compression-bandages or stockings, including any specific washing instructions. The person should also be informed of measures that keep compression bandages or stockings dry while bathing.

Conclusion

A comprehensive assessment of the person with a leg ulcer is imperative to confirm ulcer aetiology. Graded compression therapy is the definitive treatment for venous leg ulcers.

The ability to utilise compression therapy requires knowledge and skill. Implementation of a sound, evidence-based treatment plan in conjunction with the person can achieve a positive outcome.

Chapter 12
Pressure Ulcers

Jenny Prentice

Introduction

A pressure ulcer can be defined as ' … any lesion caused by unrelieved pressure resulting in damage of underlying tissue' (NPUAP 1989). Pressure ulcers are painful debilitating wounds. They are associated with significant morbidity and mortality in frail older people, people who are immobile, people who have neurological impairment, and those who are critically ill (Allman et al. 1986; Burd et al. 1992).

More than a million hospitalised patients in America develop one or more pressure ulcers per year (Young, Evans & Davis 2003), as do about 10% of all adult patients in the United Kingdom (Harding & Boyce 1998) and more than 60,000 Australians (Porter & Cooter 1999).

Pathophysiology of pressure ulcers
Overall picture

Pressure-induced tissue injury arises from a complex series of events. The main factor leading to the development of pressure ulcers is unrelieved pressure (especially over bony prominences) resulting in gross tissue deformation and occlusion of blood and lymphatic flow (Scales 1990; Bliss 1998).

Framework of chapter

This chapter discusses pressure ulcers under the following headings:

When a person is lying or sitting, pressure is unequally distributed over the skin's surface. Pressure is exerted over a smaller surface area, and can be concentrated at a particular point (such as the hip or heel). This 'point pressure' produces several deleterious effects in the skin and underlying deeper tissues—by increasing capillary permeability, increasing interstitial oedema, and blocking lymphatic and venous drainage. Over time this causes tissue ischaemia, which leads to necrosis and the formation of a pressure ulcer (Torrance 1983; Young & Dobranski 1992).

'People who have impaired sensory perception or require assistance to change their positions are at risk of developing pressure ulcers from point pressure.'

People who have intact sensory pathways reposition themselves in response to discomfort. However, people who have impaired sensory perception or those who require assistance to change their positions are at risk of developing pressure ulcers from the effects of point pressure (Exton-Smith & Sherwin 1961). The effect of applied pressure on soft tissue is determined by: (i) the intensity and duration of the pressure; and (ii) the tissue tolerance to pressure (AWMA 2001).

Capillary-closing pressures

The association between the development of pressure ulcers and capillary pressures (especially capillary-closing pressures) has been widely debated

(Feedar 1995; Wysocki & Bryant 1992). Capillary pressure readings have largely been obtained from healthy male adults, and these readings might not correlate with the capillary pressures of compromised individuals who are at risk of developing pressure ulcers (Bryant et al. 1992).

Normal capillary pressure refers to the pressure of blood flowing from arterial capillaries through the mid-capillary bed out to the venous capillary system. Capillary pressures are commonly cited as being 30–40 mm Hg in the arteriole limb, 20–25 mm Hg in the mid-capillary bed, and 10–14 mm Hg in the venous limb (Bryant et al. 1992; Krouskop 1983). Because the capillary walls are thin, blood flow through capillary loops that extend into the dermis is affected by external pressures and skin temperature (Feedar 1995).

To impede blood flow, capillary-closing pressures must exceed usual capillary pressures. Capillary-closing pressures range from 10 mm Hg to 40 mm Hg. However, this is an approximation because people with localised or systemic circulatory deficits are likely to have lower capillary pressures (Bryant et al. 1992; Krouskop 1983). Capillary-closing thresholds are also influenced by the collagen content of the dermis and auto-regulatory mechanisms of the microcirculation (Hitch 1995).

The microvasculature system can be further impaired by: (i) damage to the endothelial cells that line capillary walls; (ii) venous obstruction from venous micro-thrombi formed as a result of the clotting cascade (Michel & Gillott 1990); and (iii) reduced lymphatic vessel motility caused by tissue hypoxia leading to stasis of interstitial fluid and raised interstitial oncotic pressure (Reddy, Cochran & Krouskop 1980).

Tissue tolerance

Low-intensity pressure that is applied to tissue for a prolonged period of time causes similar tissue damage to that of high-intensity pressure applied for a short period of time (Dinsdale 1974).

The term 'tissue tolerance' refers to the integrity of the skin and its underlying supporting structures, and its ability to transmit applied pressure from the skin to the skeleton without adverse effects. Tissue tolerance is affected by many factors—including shearing force, friction, moisture, age, diabetes, nutritional status, neurological disorders, and surgery (Koziak 1961; Braden & Bergstrom 1987).

Pathophysiological changes

Sustained applied pressure produces a sequence of pathophysiological changes in soft tissue and muscle. These changes include (Bates-Jensen 1998; Bryant et al. 1992):

- blanching;
- reactive hyperaemia;
- reperfusion injury;
- non-reactive hyperaemia;
- hypoxia; and
- tissue necrosis.

Blanching

Blanching is a pale appearance of the skin as a result of temporary occlusion of blood flow and local tissue hypoxia.

Reactive hyperaemia

Reactive hyperaemia (or 'blanching erythema') is a transient red flush in the skin that occurs when pressure is relieved. It is a normal response in healthy skin, but can also be the earliest sign of pressure damage. Further tissue damage is avoidable if the pressure is relieved.

Reperfusion injury

Reperfusion injury occurs when there are repeated episodes of applied pressure to the same area. These induce further tissue hypoxia which, in turn, is aggravated by the formation of micro-thrombi.

Non-reactive hyperaemia

Non-reactive hyperaemia results from prolonged applied pressure and tissue deformation. The skin does not blanch because damaged blood vessels allow extravasated blood to leak into the surrounding tissues. The

Pathophysiological changes

This portion of the text discusses the following pathophysiological changes:

- blanching;
- reactive hyperaemia;
- reperfusion injury;
- non-reactive hyperaemia;
- hypoxia; and
- tissue necrosis.

skin is characterised by discolouration (bright, dark-red, or purple), and can feel indurated or boggy on palpation.

Hypoxia

Hypoxia occurs as a result of prolonged capillary occlusion—which deprives cells of vital oxygen and nutrients. Cell permeability increases and cellular waste cannot be processed. This leads to increased tissue oedema, tissue hypoxia, and cell death. At this stage, the tissues are unable to recover, and a pressure ulcer will form.

Tissue necrosis

Tissue necrosis (death of tissue) is the final pathophysiological stage in the formation of a pressure ulcer.

It should be noted that skin erythema over bony prominences is usually taken to be an early sign of pressure-induced tissue damage. However, necrosis of muscle and fascia might already have occurred at the bony interface (where tissue pressures are highest). The reason for this deep-tissue damage is that muscle tissue is less resistant to pressure than skin (Shea 1975).

'Skin erythema over bony prominences is an early sign of pressure-induced tissue damage ... [but] necrosis of muscle and fascia might already have occurred.'

Complications of pressure ulcers

Sepsis and osteomyelitis

The main complications associated with pressure ulcers are sepsis and osteomyelitis. Pressure ulcers breach the epidermis and can cause significant tissue damage to subcutaneous tissue, muscle, and bone. Once the protective barrier of the epidermis is lost, contamination and colonisation of the damaged tissue with cutaneous bacterial flora can occur. If local defence mechanisms are insufficient, contamination can escalate to infection. Interference with healing processes (such as angiogenesis and collagen synthesis) can then occur and aggravate the situation (Smith, Black & Black 1999; Maklebust & Sieggreen 1996).

'The main complications associated with pressure ulcers are sepsis and osteomyelitis.'

The signs of clinical infection include heat and induration of the surrounding tissues, localised oedema, fever, pain, and purulent wound drainage.

The most common causative organism of cellulitis associated with pressure ulcers is *Staphylococcus aureus*. Infection in deeper ulcers can involve a variety of organisms—including aerobic bacteria (such as *S. aureus*, *Escherichia coli*, *Pseudomonas aeruginosa*, and group A streptococci) and/or anaerobic bacteria (such as *Bacteroides fragilis*) (Smith, Black & Black 1999).

It can be difficult to diagnose osteomyelitis in patients with pressure ulcers—especially those with stage 3 or stage 4 ulcers in the pelvic region who have been receiving antibiotics (Hirshberg et al. 2000). To confirm the diagnosis of osteomyelitis, needle bone biopsy might be required (Thomas 2001).

Quality of life

Secondary complications of infection of pressure ulcers include pain, altered body image, loss of control, lack of privacy, feelings of social isolation, and decreased self-worth (Clark 2002; Wellard 2001).

Increased mortality

There is an association between pressure ulcers and increased mortality. Although the exact mechanism of this link is unclear, the fact that pressure ulcers occur most commonly in frail, elderly, and compromised patients is likely to account for the increased mortality (Thomas 2001).

Preventing pressure ulcers

All clinicians should be aware of the importance of preventing pressure ulcers when patients are admitted to (or transferred between) healthcare facilities. This can easily be overlooked if patients are admitted to acute-care facilities as emergency admissions or for same-day procedures. It is therefore important that processes are embedded in organisational policy and practice to assess the risk status of patients with respect to pressure ulcers, and to initiate clinical interventions as required.

'It is important that processes are embedded in organisational policy and practice to assess the risk status of patients.'

The majority of pressure ulcers are preventable; only a small proportion of patients will 'inevitably' develop a pressure ulcer—because of multiple risk factors or underlying diseases.

To prevent pressure ulcers, certain general strategies should be put in place. These are listed in the Box on page 196.

In addition to these general strategies listed in the Box, the following practical aspects of care should be borne in mind (Bates-Jensen 1998; Maklebust & Sieggreen 1996):

- avoid massaging bony prominences—because this exacerbates damage to the microvasculature system;
- avoid positioning a patient's knees at an angle greater than 90 degrees to the hips when sitting in a chair or wheelchair—thus reducing pressure over the ischial tuberosities (of the buttocks);
- avoid raising the bedhead higher than 30 degrees from the horizontal—thus minimising shearing force and friction over the sacro-coccygeal region ('tailbone');

General strategies for prevention

The following general strategies should be put in place to prevent pressure ulcers:

- frequent skin inspection;
- early intervention;
- alleviation of any pressure;
- increase in mobility and activity;
- reduction in shearing pressure and friction;
- reduction in skin moisture (especially incontinence);
- provision of nutritional requirements;
- implementation of repositioning regimens;
- avoidance of prolonged procedures;
- correction of any underlying conditions;
- multidisciplinary assessments; and
- patient and carer education.

ADAPTED FROM NPUAP (1992) AND AWMA (2001)

- elevate the end of the bed up to 10 degrees—to reduce slipping down the bed; and
- use bed cradles or pillows to keep bedcovers off toes and reduce heel pressures.

Risk factors for pressure ulcers

Overview of risk factors

People who are 'at risk' include those with any condition that affects mobility or activity to such an extent that they are unable to reposition themselves independently to alleviate pressure (AWMA 2001). This risk is increased if certain extrinsic and intrinsic risk factors are also present.

Extrinsic factors diminish tissue tolerance to pressure, and thus increase the risk of a pressure ulcer developing. The main extrinsic risk factors include shearing forces, friction, and moisture (AWMA 2001).

The main *intrinsic* factors include nutritional deficits, impaired oxygen delivery, increased skin temperature, and chronic illnesses (such as metastatic cancer) (AWMA 2001).

Apart from these major extrinsic and intrinsic risk factors, other predisposing factors are operative procedures longer than three hours in duration, hypovolaemia, incontinence, medications, gross obesity or low body weight, ageing skin, presence of a fracture, and previous history of a pressure ulcer (Smith, Black & Black 1999; NPUAP 1992). An individual's propensity for developing pressure ulcers increases with the number of risk factors they have (Anderson & Kvorning 1982; Stotts 1987).

Risk-assessment tools

Risk-assessment tools for pressure ulcers were first developed more than forty years ago to assist clinicians in objectively measuring the risk status of patients.

Most of these risk-assessment tools assign a numerical score to one or more risk factors. The total score then indicates the patient's status— 'no risk', 'low risk', 'medium risk', 'high risk', or 'very high risk'. Typical risk factors assessed on such assessment tools include: gender; general physical condition; body mass; skin type; mental state; sensory perception; degree of mobility and activity; continence; nutritional status; exposure to friction and shear forces; history of major surgery or trauma; and medications (Bergstrom et al. 1987; Exton-Smith & Sherwin 1961; Waterlow 1988).

Several risk-assessment tools have been developed. Of these, the Norton tool (Exton-Smith & Sherwin 1961), Braden tool (Braden & Bergstrom 1987), and Waterlow tool (Waterlow 1988) have been subjected to the most rigorous testing with respect to sensitivity, specificity, predictive value of positive and negative tests, reliability, and validity (Bridel 1993; Flanagan 1993).

Risk assessment should be conducted at certain times. These include (Crest 1998; NPUAP 1992, AWMA 2001):

- on admission to a healthcare agency (including accident and emergency departments);

- on transfer from one agency or clinical unit to another;
- following a change in the patient's health status; and
- regularly and frequently throughout an episode of patient care.

Benefits of risk-assessment tools

The benefits of using of risk-assessment tools include (Hamilton 1992; Hitch 1995):

- early identification and intervention for patients at 'high risk';
- continuity of care through improved communication and documentation; and
- reduction in inappropriate, ineffective, and unsubstantiated pressure-ulcer practices.

Irrespective of which tool is employed, the key factors in reducing the prevalence and incidence of pressure ulcers are: (i) consistent use of the tool, in conjunction with clinical judgment; and (ii) active intervention to decrease identified risks (Colburn 1990).

Risk assessment is only one component of an holistic patient assessment—which should be a multidisciplinary effort from admission to discharge (Bergstrom et al. 1987; *Lancet* 1990). As Edberg, Cerny and Stauffer (1973) have observed:

> Diagnostic acumen is not measured by the ability to recognise a pressure sore once it has developed: it is the recognition of the early warning signs of potential skin breakdown and the prevention of any further progression.

Risk-assessment tools therefore should be seen as a valuable addition to the repertoire of prevention strategies for pressure ulcers (Bethell 1994). Before adopting a risk-assessment tool, several tools should be tested to determine which is most suitable for the care context in which it is to be used (Colburn 1990).

Classification of pressure ulcers

Pressure ulcers can occur on any body part that is subject to prolonged unrelieved pressure. Most ulcers are located on the sacrum, heels, elbows, trochanters (hips) and lateral malleoli (ankles).

Pressure ulcers are classified according to the degree of observable tissue damage. Shea (1975), who first classified pressure ulcers in this manner, believed that a classification system would enhance the ability of clinicians to prevent, manage, and assess the effectiveness of treatment regimens (Shea 1975).

Several other classification systems have since been developed—most notably that of the National Pressure Ulcer Advisory Panel of America (NPUAP 1992). This system ranked tissue damage on a scale of 1–4 as described in Table 12.1 (below).

Table 12.1 NPUAP definitions of stage 1–4 pressure ulcers
AUTHOR'S PRESENTATION (ADAPTED FROM NPUAP 1992)

Stage	Definition	Other defining characteristics
1	Observable pressure-related alteration of intact skin As compared with adjacent skin (or opposite side of body), changes include one or more of the following: (i) skin-temperature change (warmth or coolness); (ii) tissue-consistency change (firm or boggy feel); (iii) sensation change (pain, itching) In lightly pigmented skin, defined area of persistent redness; in darker skin tones, persistent red or blue hues can occur	Non-blanchable erythema Affected area will not blanch when light finger pressure applied; redness of skin persists for more than thirty minutes after pressure is alleviated Pitting of skin and deepening skin tones indicate stage 1 ulcers in darker skin tones (Henderson et al. 1997).
2	Partial-thickness skin loss involving epidermis and/or dermis Ulcer is a superficial abrasion, blister, or shallow crater	Will heal in response to topical therapy and pressure relief
3	Full-thickness skin loss involving damage or necrosis of subcutaneous tissue that can extend down to (but not through) underlying fascia Ulcer is a deep crater with or without undermining of adjacent tissue	Chronic exuding ulcers Often heavily colonised with bacteria; delayed wound healing Surrounding tissue can be affected by cellulitis (Bryant et al. 1992)
4	Full-thickness skin loss with extensive destruction, tissue necrosis, or damage to muscle, bone, or supporting structures (e.g., tendon or joint capsule) Undermining and sinus tracts can occur	Exhibit similar characteristics to stage 3 ulcers Preventing osteomyelitis is paramount (Bryant et al. 1992)

Classification systems have several limitations. These relate to:

- difficulties in identifying reactive hyperaemia (non-blanchable erythema);
- difficulties in identifying stage 1 pressure ulcers in people with darkly pigmented skin;
- difficulties in accurately staging pressure ulcers in the presence of necrotic tissue;
- failure to remove necrotic tissue or eschar before proceeding with ulcer classification; and
- difficulties in staging of healing ulcers

It should be noted that staging is limited to visual observation only (NPUAP 1992, AWMA 2001).

It is important that nurses are competent in quantifying the degree of tissue loss in pressure ulcers. If nurses can accurately describe and record clinical descriptions of pressure ulcers, this facilitates communication regarding the status of an ulcer, care planning, and treatment regimens (Culley 1998; Cooper 1992).

Support surfaces
Functions and terminology
The primary functions of support surfaces are (Kenny & Rithalia 1999):

- to redistribute pressure more equitably over the total body surface area; and
- to maintain patient comfort.

The terminology used to describe support surfaces varies in different countries. Some common terms used in various countries to define the function, physical properties, and desired effects of support surfaces are described in Table 12.2 (page 201).

Types of support surfaces
Support surfaces can be grouped as 'comfort devices', 'cushions and overlays', 'replacement mattresses', and 'specialty beds' (Shipperley 1998; AWMA 2001).

Table 12.2 Terminology associated with support surfaces

AUTHOR'S PRESENTATION (ADAPTED FROM KENNEY & RITHALIA 1999; AWMA 2001; NCC-NSC 2003)

Common terms	Definition	Pressure effect on skin	Category of device
Pressure-reducing (USA)	Reduction of interface pressure (not necessarily below capillary-closing pressure)	Maximises skin contact area to reduce peak interface pressures	Static or dynamic Foam, low-air-loss surfaces, gel, fibre, air-fluidised systems
Pressure-relieving (USA)	Reduction of interface pressure (below capillary-closing pressure)	Removes pressure from a localised area of skin	Static or dynamic Heel elevators, low-air-loss, alternating air-pressure mattresses or overlays
Static-support surface (Australia)	Pressure-reducing device that does not cycle in time	Maximises skin contact area to reduce peak interface pressures	Foam, water, gel, fibre-filled devices
Dynamic-support surface (Australia)	Pressure-reducing device that cyclically changes its support	Removes pressure from a localised area of skin and redistributes pressure	Alternating air-pressure mattresses or overlays
Low-tech device (UK)	Conforming support surface	Distributes the body weight over a large area	Foam, gel, air, fibre, water, bead-filled mattresses or overlays
High-tech device (UK)	Dynamic system	Removes pressure from a localised area of skin	Alternating pressure mattresses, air-fluidised beds, low-air-loss surfaces, turning beds or frames
Constant low-pressure device (UK)	Moulds to body contours	Maximises skin contact area to reduce peak interface pressures	Foam, gel, air, fibre, water-filled mattresses or overlays, air-fluidised beds, static and powered devices
Alternating-pressure device (UK)	Inflation and deflation of mattress cells occur cyclically to create areas of high and low pressures between the body and support surface	Removes pressure from a localised area of skin and redistributes pressure	Overlays, single- or multi-layered mattress replacements

Comfort (or adjunct) devices include items such as natural sheepskins. These reduce friction and shear forces over bony prominences, wick away moisture from the skin, and are comfortable for patients to lie on (Jolley et al. 2004). Other devices in this category include heel and elbow protectors—usually made out of foam, gel, or fleece.

'Comfort devices do not reduce or relieve pressure, and they should be used only as adjunct devices to promote maintenance of intact skin.'

Comfort devices do not reduce or relieve pressure, and they should be used only as adjunct devices to promote maintenance of intact skin.

Water-filled gloves, intravenous fluid bags, and ring cushions (or donut devices) are often used as adjunct devices. The use of these devices is inappropriate because they exacerbate point pressure. They should therefore be avoided (Williams 1993; Rycroft-Malone 2001).

Foam-, fibre-, or gel-filled cushions are useful aids for people who are at low risk of developing pressure ulcers. Static-air and alternating large-cell overlays are useful for people who are at low-to-moderate risk. Replacement mattresses (such as high-density, layered- or cubed-foam, and static-air mattresses) are advocated for patients who are at moderate-to-high risk. Low-air-loss and alternating large-cell mattresses are indicated if the risk is moderate to high.

Patients who are deemed to be at high-to-very-high risk might benefit from low-air-loss or air-fluidised specialty beds (Andrychuk 1998; AWMA 2001).

Choosing support surfaces

In choosing a support surface, the aim is to 'provide the lowest level of pressure-relieving equipment which will either prevent pressure damage or assist in the healing of existing pressure damage' (Shipperley 1998).

In general, all patients who are deemed to be 'at risk' or who are 'vulnerable to pressure ulcers' should be nursed on a high-specification foam mattress with pressure-relieving properties. Patients with a 'high' or 'elevated risk' of developing pressure ulcers should be placed on an alternating or other advanced pressure-relieving support surface (NICE 2003; AWMA 2001).

Some factors to consider before purchasing or renting support surfaces are presented in the Box below.

Choosing a support surface

Some factors to consider before purchasing or renting a support surface include the following.

Patient factors
- comfort
- degree of mobility
- overall risk status
- tissue tolerance and interface pressures
- goal of care
- seating and lying needs
- hours per day on device
- pressure-ulcer history
- medical history
- presence of spinal injury

Device factors
- ability to reduce or relieve pressure
- ability to reduce shear and friction forces
- ability to reduce moisture and heat retention
- patient weight limitations
- infection-retardant properties
- fire-retardant properties
- durability and warranty
- emergency features
- maintenance requirements
- minimal interference with patient-care activities
- portability of device
- cost per day

(continued)

(continued)

Manufacturer and distributor factors
- sales and service contract
- customer service
- availability of in-service education
- product guarantees
- supporting clinical data
- therapeutic goods approval

Environmental factors
- clinical setting or home environment
- noise of device
- weight of device
- safety of device

ADAPTED FROM BERGSTROM ET AL.(1994) AND YOUNG & DOBRANSKI (1992)

Occupational therapists or physiotherapists can assist in determining the lying and seating needs of patients. Algorithms or decision-making trees for support surfaces can also be utilised (Shipperley 1998; Andrychuk 1998).

'Support surfaces should be used correctly ... care should be taken to ensure that they do not, in themselves, contribute to the development of pressure ulcers.'

Support surfaces as adjunctive aids to nursing care should be used correctly (Clark & Callum 1992), and care should be taken to ensure that they do not, in themselves, contribute to the development of pressure ulcers (Andrychuk 1998). All other preventive measures—such as skin care and positioning regimens—should also be employed to ensure that the prevalence and incidence of pressure ulcers decreases (Frantz 2004).

Adjunct devices (such as sheepskins, draw sheets, blankets, and so on) should not be used between the support surface and the patient. These can reduce the effectiveness of support surfaces.

Treatment of pressure ulcers

Conservative treatment

The overall goal of conservative treatment of pressure ulcers is to avoid the need for surgical repair. Conservative treatment is underpinned by pressure relief, modification of underlying risk factors, and topical ulcer care. Additional aspects of care that should be considered include (Andrychuk 1998):

- assessment of the patient and the ulcer;
- nutritional support;
- pain relief;
- reduction in bacterial load;
- ulcer debridement; and
- promotion of a healing environment.

    Each of these is discussed below.

Assessment of the patient and the ulcer

Patient assessment should encompass physical and mental health, pain index, social and financial status, and use of medications and other substances (McGillick 1990; Oot-Giromini 1993; James 1997). Assessment is discussed in detail in Chapter 3, 'Assessment and Documentation', page 33.

    When specifically assessing a pressure ulcer, the following aspects should be recorded (Alterescue & Alterescue 1992):

- anatomical location of the ulcer;
- number of ulcers;
- length, width, and depth;
- evidence of induration, undermining, tunnelling, or sinus tracts;
- evidence of devitalised (sloughy) or necrotic tissue;
- exudate—amount and characteristics (malodour, colour);
- degree of granulation; presence of epithelial or hypergranulation tissue;
- condition of peri-ulcer skin;

- evidence of cellulitis, infection, and osteomyelitis; and
- response to local therapies (such as dressings, debridement, and pressure relief).

Conservative treatment

This portion of the text discusses the following aspects of conservative care:
- assessment of the patient and the ulcer;
- nutritional support;
- pain relief;
- reduction in bacterial load;
- ulcer debridement; and
- promotion of a healing environment.

Nutritional support

The nutritional status of patients should be assessed in relation to their anthropometric measurements and caloric requirements, their ability to eat and absorb oral food and fluids, and whether they suffer from chronic illness, infection, or sepsis.

Reduced serum albumin and serum transferrin levels might indicate malnutrition and a need for dietary supplements (NPUAP 1992). Nutrition and healing is discussed in detail in Chapter 7, 'Nutrition and Healing', page 105.

Pain relief

Pain relief that is appropriate to the cause and site should be provided—especially before repositioning and dressing changes. Effective methods might include: intranasal sprays, nitrous oxide, oral slow-release medication, nerve blocks, or systemic analgesia.

Transcutaneous electrical nerve stimulation (TENS) is useful in some patients for localised pain relief. Relief of pressure is, in itself, a significant factor in pain relief (Krasner 1997; Szor & Bourguignon 1999).

Reduction in bacterial load

The objective of wound cleansing is to remove bacteria and surface contaminants from infected and necrotic material by irrigating the ulcer with saline or tap water. Gentle cleansing is required in a healing ulcer.

Systemic antibiotic therapy should be commenced only if there is evidence of advancing cellulitis, bacteraemia, sepsis, or osteomyelitis—or after confirmation of active infection by microbiological testing (Longe 1986; Porter & Cooter 1999).

Ulcer debridement

Healing is delayed in the presence of necrotic tissue. Debridement of non-viable tissue is therefore essential—provided that there is adequate blood supply to support healing.

'Clinicians need to be aware of the contraindications and the legal and ethical implications of debridement.'

Clinicians need to be aware of the contraindications and the legal and ethical implications of debridement (Longe 1986; Eaglestein & Falanga 1997). For further discussion on debridement, see Chapter 6, 'Wound Bed Preparation', page 89.

Promotion of a healing environment

Numerous dressing options are available for treating pressure ulcers. The most important factor is to determine which dressing from each generic group of dressings is best suited to promoting a healing environment. This depends on the site of the pressure ulcer, the degree of tissue loss, the amount of exudate, wound bio-burden, frequency of dressing changes, degree of pain and patient comfort, availability and cost, and the clinical setting. Further information on dressings can be found in Chapter 4, 'Dressings', page 51.

Topical negative-pressure therapy or vacuum-assisted closure is gaining recognition as a useful method of treating recalcitrant pressure ulcers and ulcers in patients for whom surgery is contraindicated (Cograve, West & Leonard 2002). For further discussion on topical negative-pressure therapy, see Chapter 9, 'Reconstructive Techniques', page 133.

Surgical intervention

Surgery might involve debridement, excision of bony prominences, direct closure, skin grafting, or flap reconstruction. Surgical intervention is indicated:

- to clear large or dense areas of necrosis;
- to close large tissue defects (due to delayed wound healing); and
- to treat sepsis and osteomyelitis.

The sacrum, heels, greater trochanters (hips), and ischium are the areas that most commonly require surgical intervention.

The goals of surgical intervention are (Eaglestein & Falanga 1997):

- clearance of necrotic of infected tissue (including bone);
- reduction of bacterial load;
- reduction of protein loss from the wound;
- elimination of dead space;
- replacement of soft tissue;
- skin coverage;
- reduction in pain;
- improvement in vascular supply; and
- improvement in functionality, cosmesis, and quality of life.

Before surgery is considered, patients should be carefully assessed to ensure optimal surgical and rehabilitation outcomes. They should be informed of the surgical options, potential complications, and functional outcomes (short-term and long-term) (Black & Black 1987).

Post-operative care involves minimising pressure over the operative site, observing for inadequate perfusion and other complications, instigating a rehabilitation program, and patient education to avoid ulcer recurrence (Rund 1997; Kane 1997).

Conclusion

Most pressure ulcers are preventable iatrogenic injuries of the skin and underlying tissues. The incidence and prevalence of pressure ulcers can be reduced by proper risk assessment, early intervention, and preventive strategies to relieve pressure (such as skin care, repositioning regimens, and the use of support surfaces).

The development of pressure ulcers in individuals who were deemed, on admission, to be 'not at risk' or 'at low risk' reflects on the quality of care provided within a healthcare facility.

Chapter 13

Burns

Sheila Kavanagh

Introduction

> It could be said that a burn wound and all of the subsequent events
> observed in the patient represent a continuum, without any clear
> points of separation.
>
> WILLIAMS (2002, P. 514)

Wound management in a burn-injured person is an evolving process.
Clinical practice is dictated by the pathophysiology of the burn wound,
the process of wound healing, and the factors that affect wound healing.

This chapter provides information on the care of burn wounds to
enable nurses to facilitate best outcomes for the person.

First aid

Appropriate first-aid treatment of burns can decrease the depth of the burn,
diminish pain, and facilitate speedy assessment and management.

The principles of first aid for burns are to stop the burning process
and to cool the burn wound.

Framework of the chapter

This chapter discusses burns injuries under the following headings:

- first aid (page 211);
- specialised burns treatment (page 213);
- response to burn injury (page 213);
- estimation of burn area (page 215);
- depth of burn wound (page 217); and
- burn wound management (page 218).

The wound should be cooled by placing it under cold running tap water for 20 minutes (or for 20–60 minutes in the case of chemical burns), but care should be taken to avoid hypothermia in very young and very old people (ANZBA 2004). It is often difficult to keep children's burns under cold running water without causing added distress to the child. As an alternative, cloths soaked in cold (not icy) water can be applied. However, the cloths should be changed frequently to keep them cool.

'If the first encounter with the person is within three hours of the initial burn injury, first aid should be administered.'

If the first encounter with the person is within three hours of the initial burn injury, first aid should be administered. Once the burn has been cooled, it should then be covered with clingfilm or a hydrogel dressing before the person is transported to medical assistance. This keeps the wound clean and minimises the pain that can occur if the surface of the wound is exposed to air.

Caution has to be taken when using clingfilm. It should not be used on the face (because this poses a risk of suffocation), should not be wrapped tightly around limbs (because this can restrict circulation), and should not be used extensively when the environmental temperature is high (because this can overheat the person).

Specialised burns treatment

Most people with a burn injury do not require care in a specialised burns unit. The Box below provides guidance on the criteria that can be used in assessing whether treatment in a specialised burns unit is required.

Criteria for specialised burns treatment

The following criteria are endorsed by the Australian & New Zealand Burn Association in assessing whether burns require treatment in a specialised burns unit (ANZBA 2004):

- burns greater than 10% of total body surface area (TBSA);
- burns of special areas—face, hands, feet, genitalia, perineum, and major joints;
- full-thickness burns greater than 5% of TBSA;
- electrical burns;
- chemical burns;
- burns with an associated inhalation injury;
- circumferential burns of the limbs or chest;
- burns in the very young or very old;
- burns in people with pre-existing medical disorders that could complicate management, prolong recovery, or increase mortality; and
- burns with associated trauma.

For people in rural and remote areas, digital photographic images (transmitted via email) in conjunction with telephone consultation can allow prompt cost-effective management. Video 'telemedicine' is more interactive and is a useful mechanism when the burns team wants to view the person's progress from a broader perspective.

Response to burn injury

Tissue destruction

Tissue injury is related to the coagulation of cellular protein caused by heat produced by thermal, chemical, electrical, or radiation energy (Byers & Flynn 1996). In all burn types, *duration of contact* is the major factor in determining extent and depth of the burn injury. In the case of specific burn injuries, the extent and depth of the injury is determined by:

- the temperature of the injurious agent (in the case of a heat injury); or
- the type, strength, and mechanism of action (in the case of a chemical injury); or
- the current conducted (in the case of electrical injury).

Burn wounds can be described in terms of three zones of tissue damage (Jackson 1953). The three zones are:

- the *zone of hyperaemia*—which usually recovers;
- the *zone of stasis*—which might or might not recover; and
- the *zone of coagulation* (or *necrosis*)—which is usually unsalvageable.

The fate of the zone of stasis is critical in determining the final depth and area of the burn wound, and it is therefore vitally important to understand the interventions that facilitate recovery of this zone. Impairment of blood flow in the zone of stasis can occur from shortly after the burn injury up to 48 hours post-burn (Williams 2002). If blood flow is compromised during this time, this can lead to the eventual necrosis of cells in this zone. Clinical management that can help to promote the recovery of this zone is summarised in the Box on page 215.

'In all burn types, duration of contact is the major factor in determining extent and depth of the burn injury.'

The body's local response to a burn injury includes release of local mediators, platelet aggregation, and increased capillary permeability. This is the starting point for the 'whole-of-body' response—which results in fluid shifts, plasma leakage into the tissues, electrolyte shifts, vascular stasis, and an intense inflammatory response.

Burn wound oedema

The formation of burn oedema is a complex process that involves massive fluid shifts into the interstitial space, loss of protein, and the production and release of local and systemic mediators.

Promoting recovery in the zone of stasis

Clinical management that can help to promote recovery in the vital zone of stasis includes:

- adequate cooling of the burn wound;
- prevention of hypothermia;
- covering of the burn wound;
- choosing a wound dressing to aid moist wound healing;
- using topical antimicrobial agents;
- adequate hydration and/or resuscitation for the person;
- elevation of the burnt area to minimise oedema;
- advising the person to avoid or minimise smoking; and
- management and monitoring of systemic diseases (such as diabetes).

Oedema occurs quickly, and can be significant within 2–3 hours of the injury. The amount of oedema is determined by the severity of the injury.

About 12 hours after the injury, the amount of oedema reaches its peak. This can be maintained for 48–72 hours. After this time, slow reabsorption begins.

The ability of the tissues to receive oxygen and nutrients is reduced during this time, and susceptibility to infection is increased (Williams 2002). Clinical strategies to aid recovery of the zone of stasis (see Box, above) must continue until oedema has resolved.

Estimation of burn area

The area of a burn in terms of total body surface area (TBSA) can be calculated using 3-dimensional computerised imaging. However, the most common method of calculating the area of a burn in terms of TBSA is still clinical observation in conjunction with a recording chart. There are three main methods:

- Wallace's 'rule of nines';
- Lund & Browder chart; and
- palmar method.

Each of these is discussed below.

Wallace's 'rule of nines'

In adults, Wallace's 'rule of nines' provides a quick estimation of the size of a burn. Various parts of the body are estimated as a percentage of the TBSA. The estimations are all 'multiples of 9' (see Figure 13.1, page 217).

- the anterior trunk (chest and abdomen) is counted as being 18% of TBSA;
- the posterior trunk (chest and abdomen) is counted as being 18%;
- the anterior aspect of each of the lower extremities is counted as 9%;
- the posterior aspect of each of the lower extremities is counted as 9%;
- each of the upper extremities (front and back) is counted as 9%; and
- the head and neck (front and back) is counted as 9%.

The genitalia and perineum are counted as the remaining 1% of TBSA.

Using the 'rule of nines', an estimation of the percentage of TBSA that has been burnt can then be calculated. However, this 'rule of nines' is not suitable for estimation of burn area in children and infants—for whom the Lund & Bowder chart (see below) should be used.

Lund & Browder chart

This chart (Lund & Browder 1944) is the most accurate clinical method of assessment of a burn area. The Lund & Browder chart lists each part of the body and provides the corresponding percentage of TBSA appropriate to that part of the body.

The Lund & Browder chart is more accurate than the 'rule of nines'. It is the preferred method for estimation of a burnt area in an infant or

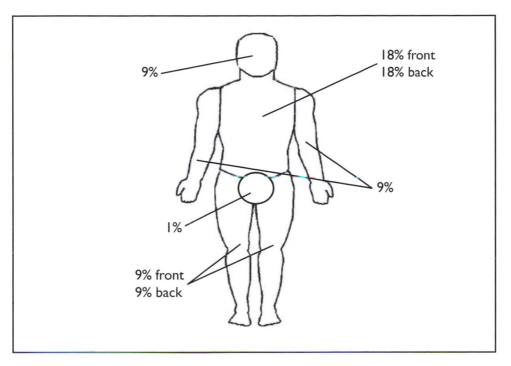

Figure 13.1 Rule of nines
AUTHOR'S PRESENTATION

child. This is because it takes into account changing proportions in TBSA with age—especially the changes in the proportions of head to body and legs to body that occur from birth to approximately 15 years of age.

Palmar method

The palmar method of assessment is commonly used for small and scattered burns. It takes the person's own palmar surface (including the fingers) as equating to approximately 0.5–1% of the person's TBSA (Carrougher 1998).

Depth of burn wound

The terminology for describing the depth of a burn has varied over time, and there is still variation among different countries. In Australia, the following terminology is used (ANZBA 2004):

- epidermal;
- superficial dermal;
- mid-dermal;
- deep dermal; and
- full thickness.

Burns can also be described as 'first degree' burns, 'second degree' burns, and so on (Williams 2002). However, this system is subject to personal interpretation. The advantage of a descriptive system ('epidermal', 'superficial dermal', and so on) is that it removes the ambiguity that can be introduced by subjective descriptions of 'degrees' of burn. This is especially important when burn wound management is being discussed on the telephone.

'Clinical observation by an experienced clinician remains the most common method of assessing burn wound depth.'

Assessment of burn depth can also be made by thermography, ultrasound, magnetic resonance imaging, light reflectance, and laser Doppler. These techniques require specialist training if reliable results are to be achieved. Clinical observation by an experienced clinician remains the most common method of assessing burn wound depth.

Burn wound management

Aims of care

The ultimate goal of all burn care is ' … to achieve wound closure in a timely fashion with minimal complications' (Carrougher 1998, p. 141). Shorter wound healing time results in better patient outcomes.

'Shorter wound healing time results in better patient outcomes.'

Factors that enable early closure to occur include appropriate wound care, good nutrition, maintenance of function, positive attitude, and cooperation from the person. Reduction of oedema, prevention of burn wound infection, and adequate analgesia also contribute to optimal outcome. Early surgical intervention is common practice in some burn centres.

The achievement of these goals involves the whole burns team. In particular, every member of the team must maintain high standards of infection control.

In summary, the aims of wound care are:

- to promote spontaneous healing;
- to prevent further tissue loss;
- to prevent infection;
- to provide optimal conditions for surgery if required;
- to be as painless as possible; and
- to be acceptable to the person's needs (in terms of employment, schooling, family responsibilities, and so on).

Burn wound management

This section of the text discusses the management of burns injuries under the following headings:

Blisters

There is no consensus as to whether burn blisters should be routinely debrided (Flannagan & Graham 2001). Factors to be considered include the size, site, and thickness of the blister. In general, small blisters can be left intact whereas larger blisters should be debrided and dressed (Williams 2002; Pankhurst & Pochkanawala 2002). However, every person should be treated as an individual.

The choice of dressings is an important consideration. For example, if film or hydrocolloid dressings are applied over intact blisters, the blisters often break during the time that the dressing is applied. On removal of the dressing at a later stage, loose blister skin might then need to be removed, possibly causing pain. The expectation of most patients and health professionals is that dressings will become less painful with time, and reduced analgesia is often administered for subsequent dressing changes (as compared with the analgesia given for the first dressing change). This combination of reduced analgesia and a potentially painful procedure can result in an unpleasant experience for the person.

'In general, small blisters can be left intact whereas larger blisters should be debrided and dressed. However, every person should be treated as an individual.'

The age of the person is another consideration. In children, blisters on the palm of the hand and sole of the foot are often left intact for 48 hours if there is no evidence of circulatory compromise. In adults, large blisters on the palm of the hand might impede function to a level that is unacceptable.

The cause of the burn injury should also be considered. In the case of chemical burns, the aspiration and debridement of blisters (ensuring that aspirate is not spilled onto surrounding skin) facilitates the removal of any remnants of the chemical agent.

Eschar

A burn eschar (or scab) should be removed at an early stage (Williams 2002). This is because an eschar:

- provides a medium for bacterial growth (and potential for burn wound sepsis);
- aggravates burn-induced immunosuppression;
- impairs nitrogen balance and wound healing;
- can impair haemostasis;
- contains toxins that can enter the circulatory system;
- can compromise limb perfusion (in circumferential burns); and
- can impair respiration (in burns of the trunk).

For these reasons, early excision of burn eschar is the 'gold standard' of care in most circumstances.

Wound cleansing

In practice, most patients are bathed or showered with tap water (Pankhurst & Pochkhanawala 2002; Carrougher 1998). The water should be run for several minutes before being used on the person to clear any stale water from the system. Some centres use mild antiseptic-impregnated sponges.

Maintaining warmth at the burn surface facilitates cell activity and oxygen delivery to the wound (Pankhurst & Pochkhanawala 2002). This can be achieved by:

- warming cleansing solutions;
- providing warm ambient temperature;
- avoiding lengthy dressing changes; and
- avoiding exposure of wet wound surfaces.

Ambulant patients with minimal wound-care needs can shower independently. For those who are non-ambulant and those with greater care needs, bathing can be undertaken with burn baths and portable shower trolleys. The Box on page 222 summarises the factors that should be taken into consideration in deciding bathing requirements.

Excessive immersion (more than 30 minutes) can cause pain and anxiety, and can lead to sodium and heat loss (Carrougher 1998).

Because wound debridement and manipulation is a significant cause of bacteraemia in people with burns (Carrougher 1998), cleansing and debridement should be careful, gentle, and minimal.

Bathing requirements

The following factors should be taken into consideration in deciding bathing requirements:

- the age of the person;
- the person's ability to lie still;
- the extent of open burn wound;
- the presence of wound infection;
- available equipment;
- available space;
- the person's need for physical therapy; and
- wounds or dressings that might benefit from soaking.

Body hair within the burn and within 2.5 cm of the wound periphery should be shaved, with the exception of the eyebrows (Carrougher 1998). Removing the hair:

- contributes to a decrease in the bacterial load on the wound surface;
- makes the application and integrity of occlusive dressings easier; and
- makes the removal of occlusive dressings easier and less painful.

Wound dressings

There is a wide variety of wound-dressing products available for the management of burn wounds. In practice, different products are suitable for some patients and some centres, and not for others.

When selecting a suitable dressing nurses should consider:

- the site, extent, and depth of the burn;
- the amount of exudate (largely determined by the depth of the wound);
- the type of first aid (for example, cooling with dirty water might have increased the risk of infection);

- the cause of the burn (for example, burns caused by organic liquids or hot oil have a high potential for infection);
- the person's ability to manage the dressing and the effect of the dressing on the person's lifestyle;
- the associated pain;
- the urgency of 'time to healing'; and
- the cost.

Available dressings include foams, hydrofibres, calcium alginates, hydrocolloids, hydrogels, polyurethane membrane-supported gels, film dressings, and silver-containing dressings. The Box below summarises the characteristics of an 'ideal' dressing.

The 'ideal' burns dressing

The 'ideal' burns dressing:
- protects the wound from physical damage and microorganisms;
- is comfortable, compliant, and durable;
- is non-toxic, non-adherent, and non-irritant;
- allows gaseous exchange;
- allows high humidity at the wound; and
- is compatible with topical therapeutic agents.

ADAPTED FROM PANKHURST & POCHKHANAWALA (2002)

Wound infection

Infection can cause further tissue death and extension of the burn wound. However, systemic antibiotics are usually used only when there is clinical evidence of an infection and positive identification of pathogenic organisms.

Anti-bacterial dressings are used in conjunction with systemic antibiotics when there is evidence of infection. Dressings for infection should:

- remove exudate;
- reduce bacterial load; and
- remove cellular debris.

In the case of a split-thickness skin graft, the purulent ooze of infection can form a physical barrier between the skin graft and the recipient bed, and can thus interfere with the 'take' of the skin graft. A combination of topical antibacterials, systemic antibiotics, and regular wound cleaning (with removal of purulent collections from beneath the skin graft) optimises graft survival.

Management of superficial (epidermal) burns

In superficial burns with no epidermal loss, a dressing is not usually required. Sunburn falls into this category. These burns can be very painful and a topical analgesic cream can be useful.

Hydrogels are now used more commonly as these products become available in first-aid kits and accident & emergency departments. This can be followed by the use of a moisturising cream when the pain has eased.

However, prevention is better than treatment, and education of the public about sun protection through the use of sunblock, sunhats, and protective clothing can help to reduce the incidence of sunburn.

Management of superficial (dermal) burns

Superficial dermal burns can be treated by a variety of wound products. These should protect the wound and encourage re-epithelialisation.

Commonly used products include polyurethane semi-permeable films, hydrocolloids, and retention dressings.

If infection is present, or if there is a high risk of infection, an antibacterial dressing should be used.

Management of partial thickness (mid-dermal and deep-dermal) burns

The management of a mid-dermal partial thickness burn injury is similar to the management of a split-thickness skin-graft donor site. The donor site should have a low risk of infection and antibacterial dressings are not normally required.

Products that might be considered for these burns include:

- hydrocolloids;
- polyurethane films;
- biologic dressings;
- biosynthetic dressings;
- alginates;
- polyurethane membrane-supported gel; and
- foams.

Temporary skin substitutes are becoming more widely used in the treatment of mid-to-deep burns. Because these products do not have any antibacterial properties, meticulous wound cleaning must be undertaken before application. Many centres administer a general anaesthetic to allow thorough cleansing to take place without undue distress to the person.

The use of retentive tape (rather than staples) to fix these substitutes eliminates the pain that is associated with staple removal.

The choice of dressing product is guided by the principles discussed previously, the availability of products, and the expertise of nurses in the use of these products. As with superficial burns, antibacterial dressings should be used in the presence or suspicion of infection.

Some facilities use cultured epithelial autograft for the management of partial-thickness burns. This product is often supplied as 'cells in suspension' because these can be available within 48 hours of a biopsy being received by the laboratory. Cells can also be grown to match the cell type of the area that has been burnt—for example, using glabrous (hair-free) skin for burns to the sole of the foot.

Management of full-thickness burns

The treatment of choice for full-thickness burns is early surgical excision of the burn and application of split-thickness skin grafts and/or skin substitutes. Until surgery is undertaken, full-thickness burn injuries are treated with antimicrobial dressings to reduce the risk of infection.

In the past, silver sulphadiazine cream and silver nitrate solution were commonly used, but there is now a wider variety of silver-containing dressings available. There are advantages and disadvantages to each of these dressings. The factors to be considered in choosing silver-containing dressings are summarised in the Box below.

Choosing silver-containing dressings

The factors to be considered in choosing silver-containing dressings include the following:

- the probable time to surgery (it is uneconomical to use expensive products if they are to be removed in a short time);
- the proximity of skin grafts or skin substitutes (creams can cause separation of substitutes or grafts);
- the presence of an escharotomy site (see below for more on this);
- access required to the wound for observation;
- the temperature of the person; and
- the availability of the product.

Management of circumferential burns

In circumferential burns, depending on the site of the burn, there is a risk of circulatory or respiratory compromise. This is especially the case in full-thickness burns, but can occur in a deep-dermal injury.

If this compromise occurs, an escharotomy must be performed. This is a longitudinal incision that runs the length of the burn. If possible, the incision should start in unburned skin and continue over into unburned skin at the distal end of the incision. There will be some bleeding from the incision and a haemostatic alginate should be used on the escharotomy incision if full excision of the eschar is to occur at another time.

'In circumferential burns there is a risk of circulatory or respiratory compromise.'

In any circumferential burn, care must be taken when applying dressings to ensure:

- that dressings are not constrictive in any way;
- that dressings allow for full assessment of neurovascular or respiratory status; and
- that the limb is elevated.

Management of burn itch

Burn itch is very common in many people who have suffered a burn injury, and is one of the most frustrating sequelae of a burn injury. The itch is usually worse at night. This results in poor sleep and diminished quality of life. Itch can last for several years.

Pharmacological options for treatment of itch include oral antihistamines, oral analgesics, topical local analgesics, and topical antihistamines. Non-pharmacological options include massage therapy, moisturising cream, pressure garments, and topical oatmeal products.

Scar management

The aim of scar management is to flatten, soften, and reduce the inflammation and redness in the burn scar. This can be achieved by a variety of modalities—including pressure therapy, massage, and the use of fixative dressings.

Pressure therapy might take the form of compression garments, individualised acrylic face masks, or support bandages. This normally continues for 12–18 months.

Conclusion

Burn wound management involves more than just wound dressings. This chapter has discussed some of the many aspects of burns management that can influence the outcome. These include appropriate first aid, bed rest, elevation, observation, reporting, and wound cleansing.

Burns of various depths require individual treatment—within the context of the person's needs. The site and size of the injury influence decision-making.

The key to good wound management is flexibility and lateral thinking.

Chapter 14
Diabetes
Tazmin Clingan

Introduction

Diabetes interferes with wound healing at several levels, and the healing of wounds in people with diabetes is often unpredictable. Hyperglycaemia alters the cellular function of fibroblasts and neutrophils—leading to greater susceptibility to infection.

The effects of diabetes on the normal inflammatory and proliferative phases of wound healing can be divided into *systemic effects* and *local effects*.

Systemic factors include:

- hyperglycaemia;
- peripheral neuropathy; and
- peripheral vascular disease.

Local factors include:

- wound infection;
- tissue hypoxia;
- repeated trauma; and
- the presence of necrotic tissue.

Framework of the chapter

This chapter discusses diabetes and wound care with an emphasis on the common problem of foot ulcers in diabetes. The chapter is arranged as follows:

Diabetes and foot ulcers

Diabetes is often associated with peripheral vascular disease and peripheral neuropathy. An otherwise trivial injury to the foot of a person who suffers from these conditions can result in an ulcer. If appropriate treatment is not implemented or if the vascular disease is too severe, the ulcer will not heal—thus increasing the risk of infection. Infection can spread into soft tissue and bone very quickly. Amputation might ultimately become necessary.

'An otherwise trivial injury to the foot can result in an ulcer.'

Foot disease in the context of diabetes is the most common cause of non-traumatic lower-limb amputation—usually as a result of unhealed foot ulceration. However, amputation is not inevitable. Many amputations can be prevented by early identification of the problem and prompt treatment by a skilled multidisciplinary team. In addition to the patient, members of the team should include a doctor, nurse, and podiatrist experienced in wound care of people with diabetes. The team should have links to a general practitioner and community nurses, and access to referral services in microbiology, radiology, and surgery (orthopaedic and vascular).

Nurses have a vital role in identifying foot ulcers and directing the person to the most appropriate care. Nurses should be aware that the people most at risk of amputation are those who have a history of previous amputation or ulceration, and those who have decreased sensation (McGill, Molyneaux & Yue 1998). Nurses must be able to recognise the presence of peripheral neuropathy and peripheral vascular disease, know how to assess the problem, and be aware that prompt action is required in a deteriorating situation. Healing the ulcer is the best method of preventing amputation.

'Healing the ulcer is the best method of preventing amputation.'

Types of foot ulcers

The two most common causes of foot ulcers in persons with diabetes are:

- peripheral neuropathy; and
- peripheral vascular disease.

In addition to purely neuropathic and ischaemic ulcers, there is a mixed group of neuro-ischaemic ulcers.

Figure 14.1 (below) shows a typical neuropathic ulcer, Figure 14.2 (page 232) shows a typical ischaemic ulcer, and Figure 14.3 (page 232) shows a typical mixed neuro-ischaemic ulcer.

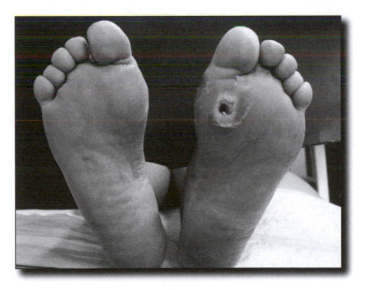

Figure 14.1 Typical neuropathic ulcer
REPRODUCED WITH PERMISSION OF DIABETES CENTRE, ROYAL PRINCE ALFRED HOSPITAL (SYDNEY)

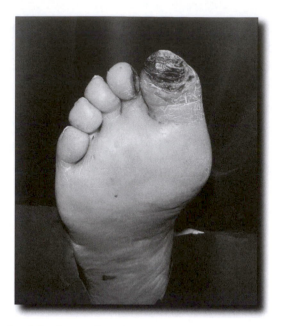

Figure 14.2 Typical ischaemic ulcer
REPRODUCED WITH PERMISSION OF DIABETES CENTRE, ROYAL PRINCE ALFRED HOSPITAL (SYDNEY)

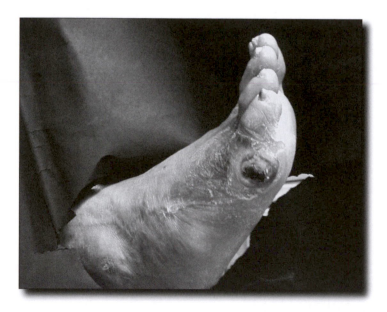

Figure 14.3 Typical mixed neuro-ischaemic ulcer
REPRODUCED WITH PERMISSION OF DIABETES CENTRE, ROYAL PRINCE ALFRED HOSPITAL (SYDNEY)

If possible, it is important to differentiate between neuropathy and vascular disease because their management differs. A *neuropathic foot* is typically warm and well perfused. Sweating is diminished, and the foot can be painless. An *ischaemic foot* is likely to be cool, pulseless, and painful.

Table 14.1 (below) summarises the characteristics of the three types of ulcers.

Table 14.1 Characteristics of neuropathic and ischaemic ulcers

AUTHOR'S PRESENTATION, REPRODUCED WITH PERMISSION OF DIABETES CENTRE, ROYAL PRINCE ALFRED HOSPITAL (SYDNEY)

	Neuropathic ulcers	**Ischaemic ulcers**	**Neuro-ischaemic ulcers**
Location	Plantar aspect of foot Areas of high pressure or trauma	Foot borders Apex of toes Dorsum of feet	Anywhere on foot
Characteristics	Callused border Punched-out appearance Can be deep Undermined edges Granulating or sloughy base	Irregular edges Can have pale, granulating, or sloughy base Can be covered with eschar	Callused border (but less callus than neuropathic ulcer) Can be deep or have undermined areas Pale-coloured granulation tissue or sloughy ulcer base
Exudate	Low-to-moderate exudate	No exudate	Low–moderate exudate
Pain	Painless	Painful	Painless
Associated clinical signs	Loss of sensation Normal pulses Warm foot Dry skin	Weak or absent foot pulses Cool foot Skin pale and shiny	Weak or absent foot pulses Loss of sensation

Peripheral neuropathy is the most common *cause* of foot ulcers in people with diabetes, whereas peripheral vascular disease is the most important factor in determining the *outcome* of ulcers.

Neuropathic ulceration

Incidence

Most foot ulcers in people with diabetes are neuropathic in origin—accounting for approximately 45–60% of all ulceration (Thomson et al. 1991).

Causes

Extrinsic injury

People with severe neuropathy are susceptible to significant injury to their feet because they lack sensation. These injuries can be caused by:

- *footwear that is too small*—the most common cause of injury, accounting for 58% of foot trauma in neuropathic ulcers (McGill, Molyneaux & Yue 2004);
- *foreign objects that have found their way into the person's footwear*—such as nails, screws, glass, and small toys; the person cannot feel these objects in his or her shoes and continues to walk, thus causing foot injury;
- *walking barefoot on sharp objects*;
- *accidents when performing 'bathroom surgery'*—such as cutting toenails, removing callus, or using chemical irritants on the foot (such as 'corn cures'); and
- *thermal injuries*—from sitting too close to heaters, using a hot-water bottle, immersing the feet in hot water, or walking barefoot on hot surfaces in summer.

Intrinsic factors

Changes in foot shape are common, especially in people with diabetes. In association with peripheral neuropathy, these changes can increase the risk of foot ulceration. These include:

- *claw toes*—callus can develop on the tips of these toes leading to ulceration; maceration and tinea pedis are common between the toes (causing interdigital ulceration);
- *prominent metatarsal heads*—callus can develop over the metatarsal heads leading to ulceration;

- *high arches*—this can increase pressure on the metatarsal heads (especially the first and fifth metatarsal heads);
- *joint stiffness*—increases the pressure on the great toe leading to ulceration; and
- *cracked (fissured) heels*—can provide an entry point for bacteria.

In all these problems, callus formation can occur. Callus is dangerous in the diabetic foot, and should be viewed as a potential pre-ulcerous lesion. Standing and walking on these insensitive pressure areas increases the thickness of callus. This can eventually break down—leading to ulceration.

'Callus is dangerous in the diabetic foot, and should be viewed as a potential pre-ulcerous lesion.'

Callus that is dark and appears to contain blood is known as 'haemorrhagic callus'. It is a warning sign that there might be an ulcer underneath the callus. This callus should be removed immediately by a podiatrist.

People with dry and cracked heels require assessment because deep cracks are a portal for infection, and this can lead to ulceration.

Assessment of peripheral neuropathy

To determine if a person has neuropathy, a clear history and careful examination are required.

There are two main syndromes of peripheral neuropathy—(i) painless (or insensate); and (ii) painful. The majority of people fit into the first category. They have lost pain sensation and therefore cannot feel injuries to their feet. This places them at extremely high risk of ulceration. The second category of people can experience burning, numbness, paraesthesia ('pins and needles'), and pain. If neuropathy is due to diabetes, the signs and symptoms are usually bilateral and equal in severity.

To assess for neuropathy, nurses should:

- examine the feet for signs of conditions that are often associated with neuropathy—such as claw toes, loss of fat padding, and excessively dry skin;
- test the person's foot sensation using a 5.07 (10 gram) monofilament (see Figure 14.4, page 236);

- test ankle reflexes (which can be diminished with neuropathy); and
- use a tuning fork or biothesiometer to determine the degree of vibration sensation (which can be reduced with neuropathy).

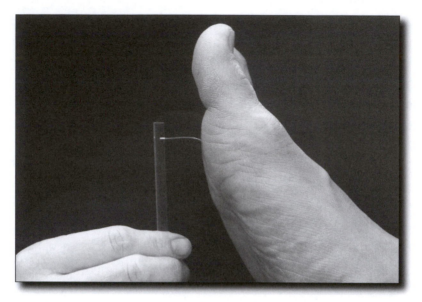

Figure 14.4 Testing sensation using a 10 g monofilament
REPRODUCED WITH PERMISSION OF DIABETES CENTRE, ROYAL PRINCE ALFRED HOSPITAL (SYDNEY)

Ischaemic ulceration

Ulceration occurring in a poorly perfused foot is rarely caused by vascular disease itself. Ulcers are usually initiated by precipitating trauma—such as knocking the foot, failure to feel pressure from ill-fitting shoes, or cracks developing in the heels. These ulcers are often painful and difficult to heal. Referral to a vascular surgeon is usually required.

Assessment

Assessment of an ischaemic ulcer includes consideration of:

- medical history;
- assessment of foot perfusion; and
- assessment of the ulcer itself.

Each of these is considered below.

Medical history

The prognosis of a vascular ulcer is dependent on the person's general health and diabetes control. Risk factors that should be assessed include:

- co-morbidities—such as nephropathy, retinopathy, and cardiovascular disease;
- poor glucose control—a glycated haemoglobin (HbA1c) of 8.0% or less is adequate for wound healing;
- smoking; and
- some medications—such as steroids.

Assessment of foot perfusion

To assess foot perfusion, nurses should:

- seek a history of ischaemic pain;
- observe for signs of reduced foot perfusion; and
- palpate for ankle and foot pulses.

  Each of these is discussed below.

History of ischaemic pain

Nurses should enquire about symptoms of *intermittent claudication* and *rest pain*.

Patients with *intermittent claudication* experience severe pain in their calf muscles on exercise (such as walking up hills or stairs). The pain is quickly alleviated by rest. Symptoms of intermittent claudication might not be experienced if the person is able to walk only a short distance. In addition, symptoms can be masked by co-existing neuropathy.

Rest pain is a burning or aching pain that occurs when the feet are elevated. Hanging the legs in a dependent position or walking to improve the blood flow relieves the pain. This can be a debilitating problem that requires surgical intervention.

Signs of reduced foot perfusion

Nurses should look for signs of reduced foot perfusion—such as poor skin integrity, absence of hair on the feet and lower leg, and thickened toenails.

Ulcers can develop under thickened toenails. Discolouration of the nail or exudate leaking from the nail can indicate that an ulcer might be present.

Palpation of pulses

Attempts should be made to palpate the dorsalis pedis artery (on the dorsum of the foot) and the posterior tibial artery (behind the ankle).

If pulses cannot be palpated, the adequacy of perfusion needs to be checked using Doppler ultrasound pressure studies, such as an ankle–brachial pressure index (ABPI). It is important to note that the ABPI can be falsely elevated in people with diabetes if vessels are calcified. In this situation, an arterial duplex scan can be performed to establish vascular supply. (For more on ABPI, see Chapter 10, page 165.)

'It is important to note that the ABPI can be falsely elevated in people with diabetes.'

Ulcer assessment

The location and characteristics of the ulcer can help identify the ulcer (see Table 14.1, page 233).

Depth is assessed using a blunt, sterile probe to explore the wound for the presence of tendon, joint capsule, bone, undermined areas, or sinus tracts. Sinus tracts are extremely common in neuropathic ulcers, but are often unnoticed. A highly exudative wound is an indication that a sinus might be present.

Infection

Infection can occur in both neuropathic and ischaemic ulcers. Infection increases risk of amputation. The people who are most susceptible to infection are those who have poorly controlled diabetes (for example, a HbA1c greater than 10%).

Signs and symptoms of infection

The 'classical' signs and symptoms of inflammation include the following:

- heat;
- swelling;

- erythema; and
- pain.

In addition to these signs and symptoms of inflammation, signs of infection can include:

- odour;
- purulent discharge; and
- lymphangitis.

These signs and symptoms can be absent in foot ulcers in people with diabetes, thus making identification of infection more difficult. Pain is diminished or absent in neuropathic ulcers (due to lack of sensation). Heat, swelling, and erythema can be diminished or absent in ischaemic and neuro-ischaemic ulcers (due to lack of blood supply).

'The signs and symptoms of inflammation can be absent in people with diabetes, thus making identification of infection more difficult.'

Other indications of infection in an ulcer are a change of colour in the ulcer base from pink (granulating) to grey–yellow (sloughy), development of sinus, undermining of edges, and exposed bone or tendon.

When assessing infection it is important to compare the left and right feet (and lower limbs) for differences.

Investigations

Wound swabs for microscopy and culture are required. Swabbing should be repeated if the wound infection does not respond to treatment within one week of treatment being commenced.

Antibiotic therapy

There is a significant risk of infection spreading rapidly in people with diabetes. Antibiotics should therefore be started empirically—rather than being withheld until a wound swab result is available.

Staphylococcus aureus is the most common organism found in these ulcers. Antibiotics that are effective against this organism should therefore be administered.

Antibiotics should be continued until the ulcer has healed. In the case of osteomyelitis (see below), antibiotics should be continued for at least three months.

Osteomyelitis

Osteomyelitis (infection of the bone) is associated with significant morbidity. An ulcer over a bony prominence is more likely to lead to osteomyelitis.

If osteomyelitis is suspected, plain X-rays, a bone scan (combined with a Technetium-labelled white-cell scan), and magnetic resonance imaging (MRI) can help to establish the diagnosis.

Management of foot ulceration

Management of foot ulcers in people with diabetes can be considered under the following headings:

- activities of daily living;
- dressings;
- reduction of pressure;
- surgery; and
- other technologies.

Each of these is considered below.

Activities of daily living

The person should not walk around on open wounds or dressings. Slippers or shoes should always be worn.

'The person should not walk around on open wounds or dressings.'

When showering, it is recommended that people with a plantar surface ulcer do not stand with the ulcer uncovered. The person can sit on a chair and use a glove or plastic bag to cover the foot. This can be removed following the shower, and the ulcer can then be cleaned and redressed immediately.

Limb elevation is not recommended with ischaemic ulcers because this can reduce blood flow and increase pain.

Management of foot ulcers

This section of the text discusses the management of foot ulcers under the following headings:

- activities of daily living (page 240);
- dressings (page 241);
- reduction of pressure (page 244);
- surgery (page 245); and
- other technologies (page 246).

Dressings

General guidelines for dressings

Exposure of the wound for lengthy periods should be avoided. Layers of dressings that occlude the wound and cause overheating (such as a peri-pads and crêpe bandages) should also be avoided. An alternative to bandaging is to use a tubular retention dressing that holds a dressing in place without adding bulk or occluding the wound.

'Exposure of the wound for lengthy periods should be avoided.'

Flexible porous tapes should be used to secure the dressing. These can be applied over the top of the dressing without occluding the wound. Occlusive paper tapes require a 'picture-frame' technique.

Dressings should be changed every 1–3 days—depending on the level of exudate and the presence of infection. A dressing should never be left on a foot ulcer for a week or more—monitoring for infection is essential, even if the manufacturer states that the dressing can be left in place for an extended period.

Protecting the wound environment from further trauma is essential. However, packing plantar foot ulcers with gauze is contraindicated. Packing with gauze causes:

- an increase in pressure, making the ulcer deeper;
- local hypoxia and death of tissue when materials are tightly packed;

- removal of viable tissue when the dressing is removed; and
- increased risk of infection due to exudate being retained in the wound.

As alternatives to gauze, dressings specifically manufactured for cavity wounds are available. These include cavity fillers and alginate ropes.

Hydrocolloids should not be used on plantar neuropathic ulcers because they lead to pressure in weight-bearing ulcers. In addition, most hydrocolloids are:

- semi-occlusive (and therefore likely to mask infection);
- prone to causing retention of wound exudate (which causes severe maceration, retards healing, and precipitates breakdown of surrounding skin); and
- contraindicated in the presence of exposed bone or tendon.

The use of topical antiseptics in chronic wounds is somewhat controversial and there are no studies that have proven the effectiveness of these in diabetic foot ulcers.

Table 14.2 (page 243) provides a summary of suggested dressings for various wound types.

Dressings for neuropathic wounds

The dressing should be cut at least 2 cm larger than the edges of the ulcer (except for alginate and hydrofibres).

Hydrogel applied to weight-bearing ulcers must be used sparingly to avoid maceration of the area surrounding the wound. Hydrogel-impregnated products assist with keeping the gel within the wound.

Soft-gelling alginates are preferable to firm-gelling alginates because they cause less pressure in weight-bearing ulcers. Alginate should be ceased if found to be dry.

Dressings for ischaemic wounds

Hydrogel should not be used on a severely ischaemic ulcer. Hydrogels work by rehydrating tissue within the ulcer. This can enlarge the wound and macerate the area around the wound if blood supply is inadequate.

Table 14.2 Dressings for diabetic ulcers of the foot

AUTHOR'S PRESENTATION, REPRODUCED WITH PERMISSION OF DIABETES CENTRE, ROYAL PRINCE ALFRED HOSPITAL (SYDNEY)

Wound type	Neuropathic	Ischaemic	Neuro-ischaemic
Granulating (low exudate)	Foam dressing	Foam dressing	Foam dressing
Granulating (medium exudate)	High-absorbent foam dressing	Foam dressing	High-absorbent foam dressing
Granulating (high exudate)	Alginate or hydrofibre (with foam dressing) OR High-absorbent pad (with or without alginate)	Highly absorbent foam dressing	Alginate or hydrofibre (with foam dressing) OR High-absorbent pad (with or without alginate)
Black eschar/ necrotic	Foam plus hydrogel OR Multi-purpose foam dressing with additives	Foam with or without hydrogel OR Non-stick dressing	Foam (with or without hydrogel) OR Non-stick dressing OR Multi-purpose foam dressing with additives
Sloughy	Foam plus alginate OR Foam plus hydrogel OR Multi-purpose foam dressing with additives (cadexomer, iodine) OR Silver foam or hydrofibre	Foam with or without hydrogel OR Non-stick dressing OR Multi-purpose foam dressing with additives OR Silver foam or hydrofibre	Foam (with or without hydrogel) OR Multi-purpose foam dressing with additives OR Silver foam or hydrofibre

Dressings that debride the wound should not be used until information regarding blood supply or permission from the person's vascular specialist is obtained. There can be inadequate perfusion to support tissue healing.

'Compression therapy should not be used with ischaemic ulcers unless advised by the person's vascular specialist.'

Compression therapy in the form of bandages or stockings should not be used with ischaemic ulcers unless advised by the person's vascular specialist.

Dressings for neuro-ischaemic wounds

The guidelines for neuropathic wounds also apply to neuro-ischaemic wounds. However, hydrogel should not be applied until the degree of ischaemia is known.

Dermal replacement dressings

Dermal replacement is an expensive dressing that contains living tissue. It can be extremely effective in promoting healing of ulcers (Bowker & Pfeiffer 2001).

Before using this dressing, blood-sugar levels should be well controlled and foot pulses palpable (or an ABPI greater than 0.7). This dressing cannot be used if deeper tissues are involved in the ulcer, or if there is evidence of necrotic debris, sinus tracts, or clinical infection.

Reduction of pressure

Reduction of pressure at the ulcer site is an essential component of treatment. Inadequate relief of pressure occurs when the person does not rest his or her foot sufficiently, or when the pressure from foot deformity is so great that even a very short period of standing, walking, or sitting in one position is enough to traumatise the ulcer.

'Reduction of pressure at the ulcer site is an essential component of treatment.'

Debridement

Removal of all visible callus, slough, and non-viable tissue by debridement is crucial to relief of pressure (Young et al. 1992). This should be performed at weekly intervals.

Some health professionals are concerned that debridement of callus will create an ulcer or increase the size of the ulcer. However, in neuropathic ulcers with good blood supply, careful debridement outweighs the risk of a minor degree of accidental trauma inflicted by the process. In contrast, caution is required with ischaemic ulceration. In these cases, debridement should be undertaken only if the ABPI is greater than 0.5. Care should be taken to ensure that the ulcer does not bleed. If the ABPI is less than 0.5, management should be conservative because there is inadequate blood supply to support normal wound healing.

Other methods to reduce pressure

Apart from debridement, there are several techniques to reduce pressure at the ulcer site. These include the following.

- Bed rest is a simple strategy, especially when the person is in hospital; but this is harder to achieve at home.
- Discarding the offending footwear is crucial. People often continue to wear the shoes that caused the ulcer, or they begin to wear other inappropriate shoes.
- Avoiding prolonged uninterrupted sitting in a chair or wheelchair is important—especially for people with peripheral neuropathy. Due to loss of sensation, patients might not move their feet in response to pressure.
- Avoiding prolonged lying in bed is also important. Bed-bound people should have total relief of pressure on their heels (even on an air flow mattress).

Other off-loading techniques are shown in Table 14.3 (page 246). These methods help to distribute pressure evenly across the whole foot. The choice of a suitable device is based on the location and characteristics of the ulcer, and the person's physical attributes and ability to comply.

Surgery

Surgery is often indicated for foot ulceration in people with diabetes—especially if ulcers fail to heal with conservative treatment.

Vascular surgery can be useful for ischaemic ulcers by facilitating revascularisation of the affected limb.

Table 14.3 Off-loading techniques

AUTHOR'S PRESENTATION, REPRODUCED WITH PERMISSION OF DIABETES CENTRE, ROYAL PRINCE ALFRED HOSPITAL (SYDNEY)

Technique	Comments
Air-flow mattresses, bed cradles, pillows, foam tunnels	Reduce pressure on diabetic ulcer in bed Prevent development of pressure areas
Felt-adhesive padding	Applied directly to skin or within post-operative shoe or footwear with adequate room to deflect pressure from ulcer Felt should be thick enough to deflect pressure from the ulcer when patient stands Usually applied by podiatrist
Half-shoe	Forefoot half-shoes reduce pressure on forefoot ulceration Heel half-shoes reduce pressure on the heel
All-purpose boot	Reduces pressure on toes
Total-contact cast	'Gold standard' for off-loading pressure in neuropathic ulceration
Pre-fabricated walking cast and aircast	Rocker sole reduces forefoot load
Custom-made orthoses and footwear	Prevent re-ulceration

Orthopaedic surgery can restore foot alignment and stability. Surgical intervention is often required to remove bony prominences due to clawed toes and prominent metatarsal heads. Surgery can also preserve the foot in the presence of infection.

Emergency limb-threatening situations often arise because treatment has been delayed. Surgical debridement of acute deep soft-tissue infections and/or removal of osteomyelitic bone is often required.

Other technologies

Newer technologies are now being applied to wound management. These include hyperbaric-oxygen therapy, vacuum-assisted closure, laser therapy, and electronic stimulation. Most of these modalities have not been validated by randomised controlled studies, but most have anecdotal evidence of their efficacy.

Conclusion

Diabetes is the most common cause of non-traumatic lower-limb amputation. However, many amputations can be prevented by early identification of the problem and prompt treatment by a skilled team. The nurse has a major role to play in this important aspect of wound care.

Chapter 15

Malignant Wounds

Wayne Naylor

Introduction

Malignant wounds—also referred to as 'fungating' wounds, lesions, or tumours—arise when cancer cells infiltrate the structures of the skin. Although this type of wound is usually associated with advanced cancer in older patients (Haisfield-Wolfe & Rund 1997), they can also occur in younger persons.

Because malignancy involves a combination of proliferative and destructive processes, malignant wounds are quite variable in appearance. A predominantly *proliferative* growth pattern produces a nodular 'fungus-shaped' or 'cauliflower-shaped' fungating lesion, whereas a *destructive* process results in an ulcerating, crater-like wound. In many cases there is a combination of both ulceration (towards the centre) and proliferative growth (particularly at the wound margin or in early nodules). Figure 15.1 (page 250) illustrates a malignant wound with both ulcerating and proliferative features.

Because of the underlying malignancy and the fact that these wounds tend to occur in terminally ill patients, healing of malignant wounds is very unlikely to occur. In most cases the wound will continue to deteriorate over time. Healing of the wound is therefore not a realistic nursing goal.

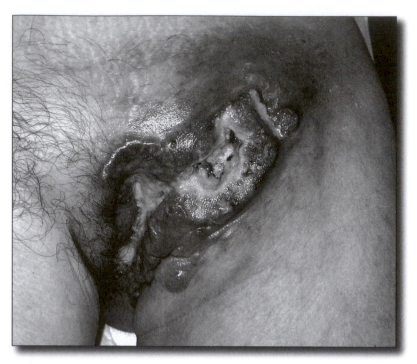

Figure 15.1 Malignant wound in the groin as a result of untreated squamous cell carcinoma of the vulva. Note deep central ulceration with proliferation at wound edges.
AUTHOR'S PHOTOGRAPH (PUBLISHED WITH PERMISSION OF PATIENT)

Malignant wound development

Although a malignant wound can arise anywhere on the body, the most common sites are the breast, head and neck, groin, and back (Thomas 1992; Wilkes et al. 2001). Cancers commonly associated with the development of malignant wounds include cancers of the breast, head and neck, kidney, lung, ovary, colon, penis, bladder, and reticulo-endothelial system (lymphoma and leukaemia) (Gallagher 1995).

A malignant wound can develop through three main mechanisms:

- from a primary skin cancer (such as squamous cell carcinoma or malignant melanoma);
- as a result of invasion of the skin by an underlying locally advanced primary or recurrent cancer (for example, breast cancer); or

- as a result of metastatic spread from a distant tumour, including implantation or 'seeding' during surgery.

Early skin infiltration often presents as discrete, non-tender skin nodules (Manning 1998). The nodules enlarge as the underlying tumour grows until it reaches a size that disrupts skin capillaries and lymph vessels. Combined with abnormal clotting and disorganised microcirculation within the tumour, the disruption of capillaries and lymph vessels causes tissue hypoxia and subsequent skin necrosis (Mortimer 1998). The result is a malignant wound.

'It is possible for a long-standing chronic wound to undergo malignant transformation— although this is less common than infiltration of the skin by malignancy.'

It is also possible for a long-standing chronic wound to undergo malignant transformation—although this is less common than infiltration of the skin by malignancy. Malignant transformation—referred to as a 'Marjolin's ulcer'—usually leads to an aggressive squamous cell carcinoma. Marjolin's ulcers occur most commonly as a result of malignant transformation of chronic burn scar ulcers, pressure ulcers, and venous leg ulcers that have been present, on average, for 25–40 years (Malheiro et al. 2001; Esther, Lamps & Schwartz 1999).

Mechanisms of formation

A malignant wound can develop through three main mechanisms:

- from a primary skin cancer (such as squamous cell carcinoma or malignant melanoma);
- as a result of invasion of the skin by an underlying locally advanced primary or recurrent cancer (for example, breast cancer); or
- as a result of metastatic spread from a distant tumour, including implantation or 'seeding' during surgery.

A wound biopsy is the only conclusive method of diagnosing a Marjolin's ulcer, but malignant change in a chronic wound should be suspected if:

- a mass appears in the wound;
- wound pain develops in a wound that was previously not painful;
- there is a change in odour of the drainage from the wound; or
- there is a change in the character, volume, or appearance of drainage.

Wound-related signs and symptoms

It is important to understand the causes of the main signs and symptoms of malignant wounds. The most frequently reported wound-related problems are malodour, exudate, pain, bleeding, and skin irritation. Each of these is discussed below.

Malodour

Malodour is predominantly a by-product of bacterial activity in the hypoxic, devitalised tissue present within the wound. Stale exudate in dressings can also be a source of malodour.

'Wound malodour is probably the most distressing feature of malignant wounds for patients—and it can also be a significant problem for family and caregivers.'

The odour associated with a malignant wound is often strong and unpleasant. It is usually persistent and can trigger gagging and vomiting reflexes (Collier 1997; Van Toller 1994). The presence of a pervasive odour can lead to feelings of embarrassment, disgust, depression, and social isolation (Van Toller 1994). The social stigma, guilt, and shame associated with a malodorous wound can also have a detrimental effect on personal relationships.

Wound malodour is probably the most distressing feature of malignant wounds for patients—and it can also be a significant problem for family and caregivers.

Indications of malignant change

Malignant change in a chronic wound should be suspected if:

- a mass appears in the wound;
- wound pain develops in a wound that was previously not painful;
- there is a change in odour of the drainage from the wound; or
- there is a change in the character, volume, or appearance of drainage.

Exudate

Heavy exudate is a common problem with malignant wounds. Patients often report problems with exudate leakage that stains their clothes and bedding—causing embarrassment, depression, and social isolation.

The high level of exudate is mainly a result of excess leakage of fluid from blood vessels. This is caused by the disorganised and highly permeable tumour vasculature, and by tumour cells secreting vascular permeability factor (Haisfield-Wolfe & Rund 1997). Tissue breakdown by bacterial proteases and inflammation associated with infection also contribute to exudate production (Collier 2000).

If an ulcerating malignant wound extends to a body cavity it can form a fistula—resulting in the discharge of corrosive or malodorous effluent. In addition, tumour necrosis as a result of cancer therapy can cause an increase in purulent exudate.

Pain

There are many causes of pain related to malignant wounds. Pain can be due to nerve and blood-vessel damage by the tumour or to exposure of dermal nerve endings from superficial ulceration.

Wound-care procedures can contribute to wound pain. For example, pain can result from dressings adhering to the wound bed or from an inappropriate cleansing technique.

Patients often complain of superficial stinging or a persistent deeper ache due to painful ulceration (Grocott 1999). Nerve damage can cause

Wound-related signs and symptoms

It is important to understand the causes of the main signs and symptoms of malignant wounds. The most frequently reported wound-related problems are:

- malodour;
- exudate;
- pain;
- bleeding;
- itching and skin irritation; and
- dressing-related problems;

Each of these is discussed in this portion of the text.

neuropathic pain—which is characterised by burning pain with intermittent sharp shooting or stabbing pains.

Bleeding

Malignant wounds bleed very easily, and sometimes profusely. This is caused by the fragile nature of blood vessels within the wound and by decreased platelet function as a result of tumour-cell activity.

Bleeding can be spontaneous or can result from trauma—particularly during dressing changes. Deep ulcerating wounds can erode a major blood vessel, thus causing profuse spontaneous bleeding that can be life-threatening. This is an extremely distressing event for the patient, his or her family, and staff.

'Deep ulcerating wounds can erode a major blood vessel, thus causing profuse spontaneous bleeding that can be life-threatening.'

Itching and skin irritation

Itching can be a chronic problem when new tumour nodules are beginning to emerge in the skin. Stretching of the skin irritates nerve endings. This causes a biochemical reaction that leads to local inflammation. Excoriation and maceration of the skin by exudate or adhesives is another source of skin irritation.

Dressing-related problems

Malignant wounds present in a variety of sizes and shapes—from small, dry necrotic skin lesions to large lesions with extensive ulceration or large protruding nodules. Figure 15.2 (below) and 15.3 (page 256) show two such lesions.

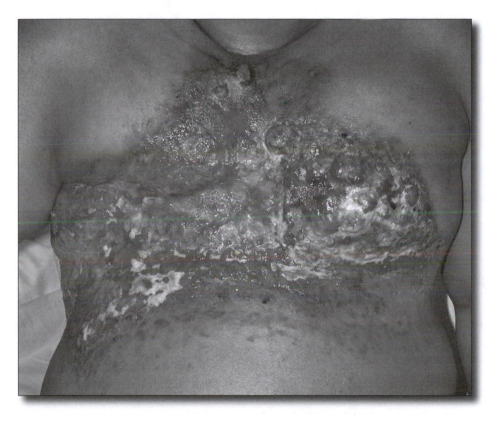

Figure 15.2 Extensive superficial ulceration of the chest wall and left breast from recurrent breast cancer previously treated with mastectomy, radiotherapy, and multiple chemotherapy regimens.
AUTHOR'S PHOTOGRAPH (PUBLISHED WITH PERMISSION OF PATIENT)

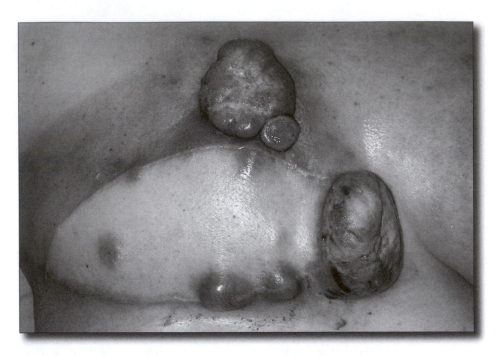

Figure 15.3 Recurrent breast cancer nodules within and surrounding a *latissimus dorsi* flap reconstruction. Note the proliferative growth giving rise to large nodular malignant wounds with central necrosis.

AUTHOR'S PHOTOGRAPH (PUBLISHED WITH PERMISSION OF PATIENT)

In view of the variety of lesions *and* the difficulties described above (malodour, exudate, bleeding, and itching), it can be difficult to choose a suitable dressing. Most of the available dressings are of an inappropriate shape and size, or do not have the required characteristics incorporated in a single product.

The wound shape and location can make dressing retention an issue. It is often necessary to avoid adhesive products—due to fragile skin, maceration from exudate, and skin stripping from frequent dressing changes. These problems are most common with heavily exuding wounds. Careful dressing selection is also necessary to avoid pain related to dressing adherence to the wound bed. It is vital to provide a cosmetically acceptable dressing that allows the patient to continue an active social life, maintain a sense of normality, and have confidence in social situations.

Management of malignant wounds

The main objective of care for a person with a malignant wound is to maintain or improve his or her quality of life by promoting comfort, confidence, and a sense of well-being—and by preventing social isolation. Management is focused on identifying realistic treatment goals, achieving effective symptom control, and preventing, as far as possible, further wound deterioration or complications.

' ... to maintain or improve quality of life by promoting comfort, confidence, and a sense of well-being.'

Assessing signs and symptoms

To manage the signs and symptoms of any condition effectively, there must be feedback from the patient on how well a management plan is working. This is of particular importance in the case of a malignant wound—because the focus of care is on improving quality of life. A comprehensive assessment identifies relevant issues and allows the nurse to work in partnership with the patient to achieve mutually agreed goals.

Assessment includes gathering information on wound characteristics and symptom severity, as well as the effect of symptoms on the patient's psychological and social status. A useful method for obtaining this type of information is patient self-report. Such self-assessment is commonly used for pain assessment, but it can be applied to other symptoms—for example, by asking patients to rate the severity of wound odour or to rate how much exudate leakage interferes with their lives (Naylor 2002).

Role of cancer therapies

Anti-cancer therapies used with palliative intent can be of significant benefit in controlling wound-related symptoms.

Radiotherapy is the most commonly used treatment. This often reduces the size of the wound—thereby decreasing exudate, bleeding, and pain.

Chemotherapy can also be effective in reducing wound size and relieving symptoms. However the response rates to palliative

Management of malignant wounds

The main objective of care for a person with a malignant wound is to maintain or improve quality of life by promoting comfort, confidence, and a sense of well-being. The following aspects of management are discussed in this portion of the text:

- assessing signs and symptoms;
- role of cancer therapies;
- management of malodour;
- management of exudate;
- management of bleeding;
- management of pain; and
- management of itching and skin irritation.

chemotherapy can be low. Hormone therapy can be of use with hormone-sensitive cancers, but can take 4–6 weeks to achieve any response.

Palliative surgery is an option in some cases to debulk or debride a large malignant wound, although problems with bleeding and underlying disease limit its usefulness. However, in selected cases, plastic surgery is a useful method of symptom control. Excision of the entire malignant wound, followed by reconstruction of the defect using flaps or skin grafts, can improve cosmesis and can provide an extended symptom-free period (Offer, Perks & Wilcock 2000).

Management of malodour

Debridement of necrotic tissue removes the medium for bacterial growth. However, the method of debridement must be carefully selected. Surgical or sharp debridement can cause excessive bleeding, and autolytic or enzymatic debridement can significantly increase exudate production (Grocott 2001).

Debridement should be undertaken only after full consideration of the benefits and the risks. It should be performed only by appropriately skilled practitioners.

Topical antibiotic therapy with 0.75–0.8% metronidazole gel kills the bacteria believed to be responsible for odour production (Newman, Allwood & Oakes 1989). Systemic metronidazole can also be effective. However, long-term therapy is often required, and this can have side-effects—including nausea, neuropathy, and alcohol intolerance. In addition, poor blood supply within the malignant wound can reduce the effectiveness of a systemic antibiotic (Thomas et al. 1998). Silver-impregnated dressings that release silver into the wound environment can also be effective in destroying odour-causing bacteria.

Another option is the use of activated-charcoal dressings. These attract and bind the molecules responsible for malodour—thus preventing the escape of odour from the local wound area (Williams 1999; Miller 1998). Sugar paste and sterile honey can also be considered.

Some honeys are active against bacteria—including antibiotic-resistant strains—and some have debriding properties. Certain honeys also contain bactericidal hydrogen peroxide and plant-derived antibacterial properties (Molan 1999; Dunford 2000). Nurses should choose a honey approved for use in wounds. The bacterial efficacy of other honeys cannot be guaranteed.

Other options include occlusive dressings that prevent odour escape, commercial deodorisers (especially those designed for use by stoma patients), and essential oils that can help to mask odours. Daily dressing changes, together with the correct disposal of soiled dressings, prevents a build-up of stale exudate.

Management of exudate

The ideal dressing choice is a product that will absorb the excess exudate while still maintaining a moist wound environment. Dressings suitable for highly exudating malignant wounds include alginate and hydrofibre dressings, foams, and those with non-adherent wound-contact layers—such as those containing silicone. These dressings can be used with a secondary absorbent pad (Grocott 1999; Pudner 1998).

If the patient is accepting of their use, continence and sanitary pads can be effective secondary dressings because they absorb large quantities of exudate and are relatively inexpensive. Wounds with a small opening but heavy exudate are amenable to management with a stomal appliance or similar device.

Reducing bacterial colonisation or infection, and reducing inflammation, will help by decreasing the associated exudate production.

Because excess exudate causes maceration, skin care is an important aspect of exudate management. Liquid skin barrier films (preferably alcohol-free) are excellent for skin protection. Alternatively, the wound can be 'framed' with a thin hydrocolloid sheet. Skin wafers, such as those used in stomal therapy, are preferable to wound hydrocolloids—because they repel exudate rather than absorb it. Adhesive dressings or tape can be fixed to the hydrocolloid frame to prevent skin stripping.

Management of bleeding

Several simple measures can be taken to reduce bleeding from a malignant wound. These include using non-adherent dressings, cleansing by irrigation, and administration of oral antifibrinolytics (such as tranexamic acid).

'If the wound is actively bleeding, management depends on the rate of blood loss.'

If the wound is actively bleeding, management depends on the rate of blood loss.

For slow oozing from capillaries, sucralfate paste or an alginate can be applied (Thomas, Vowden & Newton 1998; Emflorgo 1998). Because alginates have been reported to cause bleeding in fragile tumours, caution is advised in their use (Grocott 1998).

Moderate-to-heavy bleeding might respond to local pressure, topical haemostats, topical adrenaline, or topical tranexamic acid (the last two under medical supervision). Caution is advised with adrenaline—because overuse can cause ischaemic necrosis. Cautery or ligation by a surgeon might be necessary for heavy bleeding that will not stop.

If a major blood vessel is eroded and massive exsanguination occurs, the nurse should stay with the patient and call for assistance. The patient might need sedation if distressed—with morphine (intravenously, intramuscularly, or subcutaneously) and/or midazolam (subcutaneously). Local pressure should be applied, together with packing to the bleeding point. Nurses should monitor the patient's vital signs and, depending on prognosis, should consider arranging for a blood cross-match sample to be taken.

In some cases, it is advisable to have a strategy in place for a possible catastrophic event—for example, if the patient has a deep eroding wound

'It is advisable to have a strategy in place for a possible catastrophic event ... especially when managing patients in the community.'

in the groin or neck overlying major blood vessels. This is especially so when managing patients in the community. The patient and his or her carers should be advised how to develop an action plan to deal with a major bleed. A supply of dark towels is recommended because these can be used to soak up blood without having the dramatic visual impact of fresh blood on light-coloured towels. Easily accessible emergency contact numbers and insurance to cover ambulance trips is also advised.

Management of pain

Most patients with a malignant wound require regular analgesic medications. These should be prescribed according to the World Health Organization guidelines for the control of cancer pain (WHO 1996).

Painful dressing changes can be ameliorated by pre-medicating the patient with a short-acting opioid, by administering a booster dose of the patient's usual medication, or by using nitrous oxide gas.

Maintaining a moist wound environment and using non-adherent dressings reduces the pain associated with dressing adherence, and also protects exposed nerve endings. Less-frequent dressing changes reduce the incidence of procedural pain.

Adjunctive therapies that can help to reduce pain or alter the response to pain, particularly with anxious and stressed patients, include relaxation, distraction, and visualisation (Downing 1999).

There is growing evidence that topically applied opioids can provide effective analgesia for painful ulcerating wounds (Grocott 2000; Twillman et al. 1999; Krajnik & Zylicz 1997; Back & Finlay 1995; Stein 1995). Treatment is usually with a mixture of morphine (or diamorphine) and a hydrogel to produce a 0.1% w/w solution (1 mg of morphine per 1 gram of hydrogel). Metronidazole gel has also been used as a carrier for the opioid to provide combined pain and odour control (Flock, Gibbs & Sykes 2000; Grocott 2000).

Management of itching and skin irritation

Applying hydrogel sheets can produce a cooling effect on itching skin. The hydrogel can be covered with a semi-permeable film to prevent dehydration. Aqueous cream with menthol is a simple option that has a cooling and soothing effect while also moisturising the skin. This cream can be easily made by a pharmacy and applied to itchy areas 2–3 times a day, or as necessary (Naylor, Laverty & Mallett 2001). Transcutaneous electrical nerve stimulation (TENS) has also been reported as being effective in relieving itching (Grocott 2000).

Conclusion

This chapter has not addressed the many complex psychological and social problems associated with malignant wounds, but the chapter has attempted to provide some practical solutions to the main symptoms and problems related to these wounds. Effective wound management that addresses the symptoms and problems of most concern to the patient will undoubtedly help in reducing psychological and social distress. For example; controlling malodour and exudate reduces feelings of embarrassment and allows the patient to continue normal social interactions—such as meeting with friends and family, or enjoying an outing to a public place.

The nursing management of these wounds is difficult and challenging. However, nurses who undertake comprehensive assessment and careful planning—together with careful consideration of the patient's opinions and a hint of creativity—will usually discover a successful solution.

Chapter 16

Draining Wounds, Fistulae, and Peristomal Wounds

Keryln Carville

Introduction

Draining wounds, fistulae, and peristomal wounds present challenges to nurses and can cause significant concern to patients and their carers. The management of these wounds can be complicated—depending on the individual patient, the wound, the resources available, and the skill of the nurse.

Draining wounds

Wound exudate and moist wound-healing

Wound exudate is a pathophysiological response to tissue trauma or inflammation. It can present as interstitial fluid, a seroma, a haematoma, pus, or drainage of fluids from bodily organs.

Winter's (1962) research into the effects of moisture in promoting re-epithelialisation in wounds inspired increased interest in the nature and role of wound exudate. As a result of Winter's research, moist wound-healing became an important principle of modern wound management.

Framework of the chapter

This chapter discusses draining wounds, fistulae, and peristomal wounds under the following headings:

However, recent research has revealed differences in the composition of exudate in acute and chronic wounds (Wyscoki 1996; Parnham 2002).

'There is a growing appreciation that too much exudate can be as detrimental as too little.'

Biochemical investigations into wound fluid have demonstrated that an increase in proteases in chronic wounds can, in fact, hinder wound healing (Ovington 2002). The concept of 'moisture balance' has now become of central importance in wound management, and there is a growing appreciation that too much exudate can be as detrimental as too little.

Definition and aetiology of sinus wounds

A sinus wound is a deficit or a tract that connects the epidermis to the underlying subcutaneous tissues. The wound can be associated with undermining cavity formation or separation along fascial planes within the tissues. Such undermining can be superficial or deep.

In wounds that are healing by secondary intention, a sinus can form if the wound extends into the dermis or deeper tissues. A sinus can also be created surgically to drain a fluid collection. Such wounds can also be associated with complications in wound healing—such as dehiscence, haematoma, or inhibited healing in a drainage-tube site.

Assessment of sinus wounds

Comprehensive assessment can identify the dimensions of a superficial sinus, but a sinogram might be required when extensive tracking is suspected. A sinogram can help to determine the direction and extent of the sinus.

Management of sinus wounds

The aims of management are to facilitate healing from the base of the wound and to maintain moisture balance—while avoiding abscess formation or fluid collections in the tissues.

Large collections of fluid are best allowed to drain freely into dressings or drainage appliances.

'The aims of management are to facilitate healing from the base of the wound and to maintain moisture balance.'

Separations along fascial planes should not be packed because this can cause further separation along the tissue plane. In these cases, the goal is to facilitate wound contraction and adherence of the tissues along the fascial plane. Support garments or peri-wound strapping facilitate wound contraction and fascial plane attachment.

Wound packing might be indicated to promote granulation and controlled wound closure. The sinus should be packed lightly to avoid compression of granulation tissue. All dressing products used to pack a wound should be capable of being retrieved completely or flushed freely from the wound.

Table 16.1 (page 266) lists some primary dressings that can be used to pack a sinus. A suitable secondary dressing should then be chosen, subject to the anticipated amount of exudate.

Table 16.1 Dressings for sinus packing
AUTHOR'S PRESENTATION

Low-to-moderate exudate	Moderate-to-high exudate
hydrogels (amorphous/gel-impregnated gauzes)	hydrofibre ribbon
hydrocolloid wound pastes	hydrocolloid wound powder
calcium alginate rope or ribbon	calcium alginate ribbon or rope
hydrofibre ribbon	foam cavity fillers or expanding foam agents
ribbon gauze products (impregnated with physiological/hypertonic saline or petrolatum agents)	capillary wicking dressings

For free-draining wounds, highly absorbent dressings or ostomy and wound-management appliances (of which there is a wide variety) are preferred. The use of appliances is discussed below (see 'Fistula management', page 267).

The maintenance of moisture balance in a wound is essential for optimal healing. Excessive wound drainage has the potential to compromise a patient's general health by causing fluid, electrolyte, and nutritional deficits (Ovington 2002). Uncontrolled wound drainage compromises peri-wound skin integrity and increases the risk of infection. Protection of peri-wound skin and containment of large amounts of wound exudate are discussed below (see 'Fistula management', page 267).

Drainage tubes

Drainage tubes are inserted into the tissues or a body cavity for various reasons. These include (Brozenec 1985):

- to drain an abscessed or contaminated cavity;
- to facilitate the healing of an insecure intra-abdominal wound;
- to decrease the risk of peritonitis; and
- to avoid anticipated accumulation of secretions (for example, if surgery has involved extensive dissection).

There is a variety of drainage tubes. These include: (i) capillary drains (corrugated or portex drains); (ii) percutaneous tubes (percutaneous biliary or nephrostomy tubes); and (iii) drains connected to negative-pressure systems.

The principles of management for drainage devices include:

- observation of the tube to ensure patency and security;

- identification of the volume and type of exudate or effluent; and

- assessment of signs and symptoms that might indicate complications (such as blockage, dislodgement, infection, or damage to the peri-tubular skin).

Fistulae

Definition, causes, and types

A fistula is an abnormal tract between one viscus (or hollow organ) and another, or between one viscus (or hollow organ) and the skin (Gray & Jacobson 2002).

A fistula can occur as a result of (Carville 2001):

- congenital abnormality;

- obstruction (causing rupture of the viscus);

- chronic disease (such as Crohn's disease);

- trauma;

- radiotherapy; and

- surgery.

A 'low-output' fistula has fluid output of less than 500 mL in 24 hours. Fistulae are termed 'high output' when the volume of fluid exceeds 500 mL in 24 hours (Doughty & Broadwell Jackson 1993).

Depending on the organ involved, fistulae have different names. The terms used are listed in Table 16.2 (page 268).

Fistula management

A fistula can lead to significantly increased morbidity and mortality (Bryant 1992). As with all wounds, the care of a person with a fistula

Table 16.2 Names of fistulae

AUTHOR'S PRESENTATION

Name of fistula	Organs involved
Vesicovaginal fistula	bladder and vagina
Vesicocolonic fistula	bladder and large intestine
Enterovesical fistula	small intestine and bladder
Vesicocutaneous fistula	bladder and skin
Enterocutaneous fistula	small intestine and skin
Colocutaneous fistula	large intestine and skin
Enterocolonic fistula	small intestine and large intestine
Rectovaginal fistula	rectum and vagina
Biliary-cutaneous fistula	common bile duct and skin
Pancreatico-cutaneous fistula	pancreas and skin
Cutaneo-oesophageal fistula	skin and oesophagus

requires a multidisciplinary collaborative approach to assessment and management.

Fistula management involves the following (Carville 2001):

- comprehensive assessment of the patient, the wound, and the healing environment;
- fluid and electrolyte replacement;
- nutritional supplementation;
- prevention and management of infection;
- containment of effluent, exudate, and odour;
- maintenance of peri-fistular skin integrity; and
- optimisation of the person's quality of life.

Each of these is discussed below.

Comprehensive assessment

Following a clinical examination, laboratory and radiological investigations should be undertaken to confirm the existence of the fistula, to establish its aetiology, and to ascertain any metabolic or nutritional imbalance.

Following a comprehensive assessment, the priority of specific treatment interventions can be established. The goals are:

- surgical closure or spontaneous closure of the fistula tract; and
- correction of metabolic or nutritional deficits.

Fistula management

This section of the text discusses fistula management under the following headings:

- comprehensive assessment (page 269);
- fluid and electrolyte replacement (page 269);
- nutritional supplementation (page 270);
- prevention and management of infection (page 271);
- maintenance of peri-fistular skin integrity (page 271);
- containment of effluent, exudate, and odour (page 274); and
- optimisation of the person's quality of life (page 275).

Fluid and electrolyte replacement

To maintain fluid and electrolyte balance, it is essential to assess and monitor patients who have a fistula. Loss of fluids and electrolytes can lead to hypovolaemia and circulatory failure (Bryant 1992).

'Loss of fluids and electrolytes can lead to hypovolaemia and circulatory failure.'

The nature and potential volume of secretions depend on the type of fistula. On average, 7000–8000 mL of fluid are secreted into the gastrointestinal tract every 24 hours. Of this, only 50–200 mL are excreted in faeces; the rest is reabsorbed (Mattson Porth 1986). Table 16.3 (page 270) shows the potential volume and pH of fluid that can be lost from various gastrointestinal fistulae.

Table 16.3 Potential fluid loss from gastrointestinal fistulae
AUTHOR'S PRESENTATION ADAPTED FROM MATTSON PORTH (1986) AND BRYANT (1992)

Source	Volume (mL/24 hrs)	pH
Saliva	1000–1200	slightly acidic to slightly alkaline (6.5–7.5)
Stomach	2000–3000	acidic
Pancreas	700–1200	alkaline
Bile	500–1200	alkaline
Small intestine	2000–3000	alkaline
Colon	50–200	alkaline

Nutritional supplementation

Good nutrition and hydration are essential for well-being and healing. Nutritional fluid replacement in a person with a fistula depends on the patient's health status and the site of the fistula. This fluid replacement can be administered orally, enterally, or parenterally.

People with high output or a fistula situated high in the gastrointestinal tract usually require total parental nutrition to sustain their nutritional requirements. Secretions lost from a high gastrointestinal fistula can sometimes be re-fed via the jejunum to restore the fluid, electrolytes, and digestive enzymes that were secreted. Jejunal re-feeding involves the collection and straining of fistula effluent and re-feeding via a jejunostomy tube. Optimal hygiene and infection-control precautions are necessary when performing this procedure.

'People with high output or a fistula situated high in the gastrointestinal tract usually require total parental nutrition to sustain their nutritional requirements.'

Enteral supplementation via a gastrostomy tube is frequently used for buccal, oropharyngeal, and oesophageal fistulae. Enteral supplementation via a jejunostomy tube can be used for a low-output gastric, duodenal, or proximal jejunal fistula.

Prevention and management of infection

In persons with enteric fistulae, sepsis is associated with high mortality (Bryant 1992). Intensive medical management of infection is therefore required. This usually involves the drainage of collections and the administration of parenteral antibiotics.

The risk of secondary infections can be minimised with good nutrition, optimal wound management, and careful infection control.

Maintenance of skin integrity

The management of complex draining wounds requires expertise. In many cases, creative approaches to wound management are required.

The old adage 'pack a sinus, but drain a fistula' remains a prudent principle of management. A considerable volume of aspirate or effluent can drain from some organs of the gastrointestinal tract, and this fluid can compromise the integrity of peri-fistular skin. Maceration and subsequent ulceration of the skin can occur rapidly— especially in the presence of highly acidic or alkaline secretions.

'The old adage "pack a sinus, but drain a fistula" remains a prudent principle of management.'

The efficient containment of secretions and effluent by ostomy or wound-management appliances reduces this risk. In addition, there is a wide variety of skin-protective agents available for use.

Skin protective agents come in the form of:

- films;
- pastes;
- powders;
- adhesive skin barriers; and
- creams and ointments.

Each of these is discussed below.

Protective films

Protective films are applied to the peri-fistular or peri-stomal skin when a waterproof barrier is required. Protective films are also used to inhibit skin damage that can occur on removal of adhesive appliances or tapes.

Skin-protective agents

This section of the text discusses skin-protective agents under the following headings:

- films (page 271);
- pastes (page 272);
- powders (page 272);
- adhesive skin barriers (page 273); and
- creams and ointments (page 273).

The films are composed of alcohol or hydrocarbon-based solutions of 'plastics' that leave a protective film coating on the skin (Boyle, Fahl & O'Brien 1993). When the skin is denuded, alcohol-free agents are preferred because they can be applied without discomfort. These agents are available as single-use wipes, multi-application paint-on solutions, or sprays.

Protective barrier pastes

Protective barrier pastes contain some of the agents used in protective films and hydrocolloid skin barriers. The pastes are used for skin protection and to fill skin creases (and level skin surfaces) before the application of ostomy or wound-management appliances.

These 'ostomy' protective barrier pastes should not be confused with wound hydrocolloid pastes, which are used as cavity-filling agents. Some protective barrier pastes contain alcohol, and the application of protective barrier pastes (which contain alcohol) on denuded skin can cause stinging. These are best avoided; alcohol-free agents are preferable.

Because they are extremely 'tacky' to touch, the use of a dampened gloved finger or spatula simplifies the application of these pastes.

Protective skin-barrier powders

Protective skin-barrier powders are usually composed of carmellose sodium, pectin, and gelatin products or sterculia gum (karaya gum powder). These powders provide a protective barrier on denuded skin and absorb small amounts of exudate.

Excessive use of these agents can interfere with appliance adhesion. Excess powder should be dusted off the skin before adhesive appliances are applied.

Adhesive hydrocolloid skin barriers

Adhesive hydrocolloid skin barriers have been widely used in the management of stomas and draining wounds since the 1960s, and these agents have been incorporated into the design of many commercially available ostomy and wound-management appliances.

Hydrocolloid skin barriers come in various-sized sheets, ring shapes, and strip shapes. These products are composed of various absorptive agents—including carmellose sodium, pectin, and gelatin. The products are applied directly to the surrounding skin to protect (or level) skin surfaces. These agents are also incorporated into the skin-contact surfaces of adhesive ostomy or wound-management appliances.

Liquid skin-barrier *cement* is a relatively long-lasting adhesive skin-protective agent that can be used to protect skin at high risk of maceration. It can be used to adhere appliances that are otherwise non-adherent, or to provide increased adhesive properties if required.

Creams and ointments

There is a vast array of commercial *creams and ointments* to provide skin protection against maceration. Water-miscible products (that is, products that mix readily with water) provide minimal protection, but are more easily removed.

Emollient products are intended to provide a more durable protection, but all traces of previously used product should be removed before a fresh application because a build-up of remnant emollients can promote the growth of pathogens.

'All traces of previously used product should be removed before a fresh application because a build-up of remnant emollients can promote the growth of pathogens.'

Water-miscible and emollient products can inhibit the application of adhesive appliances. However, recent product developments have overcome some of these difficulties.

Containment of secretions, effluent, and odour

The maintenance of skin integrity requires the efficient control of wound or fistula drainage and associated odour in a cost-effective manner. Absorbent dressings are preferred for low levels of exudate or very low fistula output, but they are generally ineffective in containing larger volumes of draining exudate or effluent. Moreover, if there is a need for frequent dressing changes, this leads to patient fatigue, compromises skin integrity and patient comfort, and is not cost-effective. Alternatively, an appropriate ostomy or wound-management appliance can eliminate these concerns and can facilitate accurate observation and measurement of wound drainage.

There is a vast assortment of ostomy and wound-management appliances available. These products come in one-piece or two-piece systems, and some incorporate access ports into their design. Drainable appliances are preferred for the care of patients with draining wounds when frequent emptying is necessary. Small closed appliances or paediatric drainable appliances are alternatives when exudate levels are low or when aesthetic considerations are a high priority.

Ostomy or wound-management appliances are made of transparent or opaque materials and incorporate flat or convex skin barriers that contour to skin surfaces. Most appliances designed for fistulae or stomas of the gastrointestinal tract also incorporate a charcoal filter in their design—which allows the passage and deodorisation of flatus.

The selection of an appropriate appliance is largely dependent on:

- patient preference and the patient's ability to be self-caring;
- the anatomical site and the skin surface contours involved; and
- the anticipated volume and type of drainage.

Urostomy appliances have a non-return valve and a tap outlet. These are favoured for urine or highly enzymatic fluids (such as pancreatic or biliary fluids) because they prevent back-flow or pooling of fluids against the fistula aperture and immediate peri-fistula skin. Two-piece appliances or those with access ports are used if frequent access to the wound is required. Appliances for high-output fistulae should be capable of being connected to a secondary or night-drainage system to avoid the need for frequent emptying—especially during the night when rest is important.

If the available commercial appliances are not appropriate to manage a wound of a particular size or shape, an appliance can be constructed from plastic bags, double-sided adhesive tape, and skin-barrier hydrocolloid sheets. So-called 'parcel' dressings are of this type. They are useful when the wound dressing is attended frequently—such as during mechanical debridement. Parcel dressings are constructed from a sheet of plastic, rather than a plastic bag. Double-sided adhesive tape is used to adhere the plastic sheet or bag to the non-adhesive layer of the hydrocolloid skin barrier. A pattern template of the wound shape is drawn and transposed onto the hydrocolloid skin-barrier backing paper. The wound shape is cut out and the constructed appliance is adhered to the peri-wound skin in the same manner as that employed with a commercial appliance. The plastic envelope is wrapped around the wound and secured with adhesive tape or clips.

Optimisation of quality of life

The nursing management of a person with a fistula (or any draining wound) should be geared towards optimising quality of life and comfort. Severely ulcerated peri-wound skin can be extremely painful. The physical and psychological distress caused by leaking malodorous effluent is significant. In addition, fatigue associated with frequent dressing changes is debilitating.

'The nursing management of a person with a fistula (or any draining wound) should be geared towards optimising quality of life and comfort.'

The explicit and implicit costs associated with the care of a person with a fistula or a complex draining wound are difficult to calculate, but they are significant. Moreover, they are exacerbated by ineffectual management. The goals of care should be established with regard to the problems that exist and those that can be anticipated.

Pictorial case study

Appendix 16.1 (page 279) presents a pictorial case study illustrating the use of some of the skin-protective agents and appliances discussed above.

Negative-pressure vacuum-assisted wound closure

In recent years there has been an evolving appreciation of the benefits of negative-pressure vacuum-assisted wound closure in the management of various types of complex draining wounds (Argenta & Morykwas 1997; Hardcastle 1998). Negative-pressure vacuum-assisted wound closure is discussed in detail in Chapter 9, 'Reconstructive Techniques', page 142.

Peristomal wounds

Frequency and causes

The rate of peristomal skin complications ranges from 18% to 55% (Ratliff & Donovan 2001). These complications can result from:

- trauma;
- post-operative complications (such as mucocutaneous separation or infection);
- disease processes (such as Crohn's disease);
- inflammatory and infective processes (such as pyoderma gangrenosum); and
- chemical dermatitis (from ill-fitting or leaking appliances).

Chemical trauma or irritant dermatitis from ill-fitting or leaking appliances is perhaps the commonest cause of peristomal skin trauma. Unprotected peristomal skin, especially around a urostomy or ileostomy, is at risk of ulceration.

Bacterial infections are a relatively uncommon cause of peristomal skin problems. However, fungal infections (such as *Candida*) can be problematic, and require appropriate antifungal treatment.

Mucocutaneous separation

The term 'mucocutaneous separation' is used to describe post-operative dehiscence at the border between the stomal mucosa and the surrounding skin. The separation can be partial (which results in a local defect) or it can be circumferential (leading to retraction of the gut opening below the skin surface).

Mucocutaneous separation results from poor surgical technique or from complications such as infection, haematoma, abdominal distension, or obesity. Most partial mucocutaneous wounds are allowed to heal by secondary intention—although a surgical review is warranted when complete separation occurs. Surgical review is also indicated if partial separation occurs in the immediate post-operative phase—when resuturing might be the preferred option.

Superficial mucocutaneous wounds respond well to the application of skin-barrier powders (see this chapter, page 272). These are covered by skin-barrier pastes, rings, or hydrocolloid skin-barrier sheets to ensure a secure surface for attaching an ostomy appliance.

In cases of a deep defect or sinus tracking, absorbent calcium alginate or hydrofibre ropes (or ribbons) can be used to fill the cavity lightly. These products can be covered and sealed with skin-barrier agents before applying an ostomy appliance.

In the treatment of these wounds it is best to avoid moisture-donating cavity-filling agents (such as hydrogels) because these products compromise the wearing of ostomy appliances.

Conclusion

The management of fistulae, draining wounds, and peristomal wounds can present considerable challenges for wound-care nurses. However, these challenges can be overcome with a comprehensive and collaborative approach to assessment and management, and a good knowledge of the range of dressings and devices available.

Appendix 16.1

Pictorial case study

The presence of multiple wounds, stomas, or fistulae can be a particular management challenge—especially when these structures are in close apposition. The following pictorial case study demonstrates the use of skin-protective agents and appliances (as discussed in the text of the chapter, beginning on page 271).

The case study involves the management of a patient with an ileostomy, a colostomy, and two enterocutaneous fistulae—which drained from a dehisced abdominal suture line. Both the ileostomy and the colostomy were active—the latter due to the presence of an internal enterocolonic fistula. The two enterocutaneous fistulae that were situated in the incision site were flush to the skin surface and drained large volumes of purulent faecal fluid. The active colostomy was retracted to well below the skin surface, and leakage was a significant problem.

The primary goals of care were: (i) to contain effluent, exudate, and odour; (ii) to optimise skin integrity; and (iii) to improve the patient's quality of life.

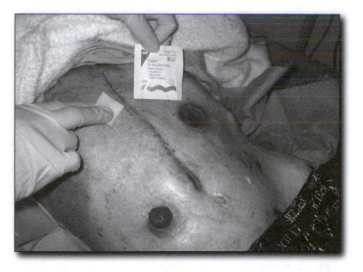

Figure 16.1 Application of protective skin film around fistulae and stomas.

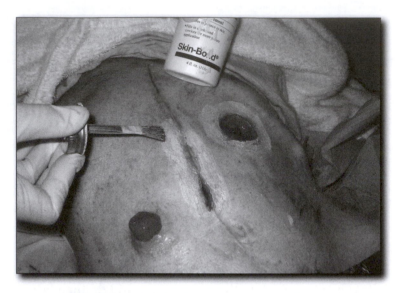

Figure 16.2 Application of skin-barrier cement for added skin protection around flush fistulae and retracted colostomy.

AUTHOR'S PRESENTATION

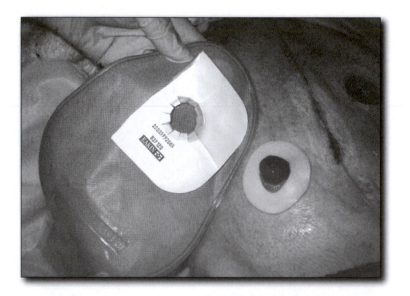

Figure 16.3 Skin-barrier seals or rings are applied to peristomal skin around ileostomy for added security, and the ostomy appliance is trimmed to accommodate the adjacent fistula appliance.

AUTHOR'S PRESENTATION

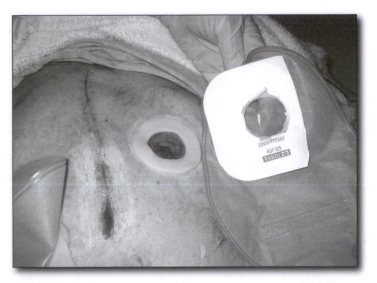

Figure 16.4 Skin-barrier seals are applied to peristomal skin around the retracted colostomy to provide a degree of convexity to facilitate drainage and security. The ostomy appliance is trimmed to accommodate the adjacent fistula appliance.

AUTHOR'S PRESENTATION

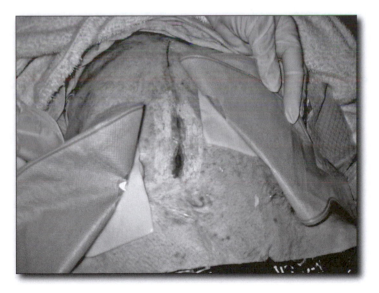

Figure 16.5 The trimmed ostomy appliances are applied to the stomas.

AUTHOR'S PRESENTATION

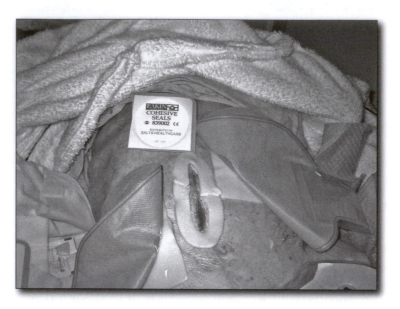

Figure 16.6 The skin-barrier seals are shaped to fit the peri-fistular skin.

AUTHOR'S PRESENTATION

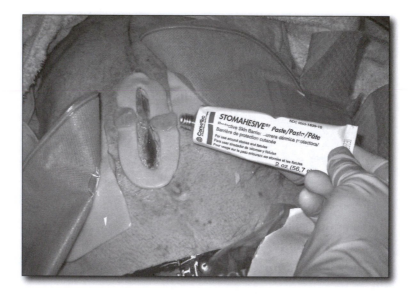

Figure 16.7 Ostomy paste is used to fill joins in seals and creases in adjacent skin.

AUTHOR'S PRESENTATION

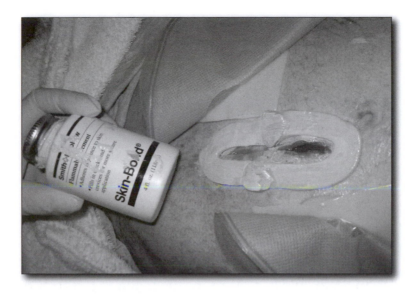

Figure 16.8 Skin-barrier cement is applied to seals to aid adhesive security and increase durability.

AUTHOR'S PRESENTATION

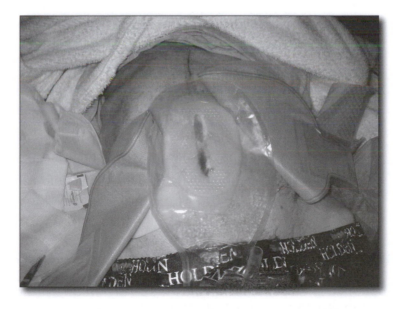

Figure 16.9 Fistula appliance is applied.

AUTHOR'S PRESENTATION

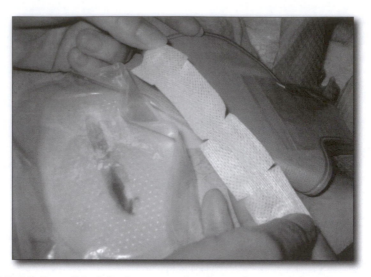

Figure 16.10 Small 'nicks' are cut in the edges of the fixation tape to increase conformability of tape when it is applied to appliance edges and skin surfaces.

AUTHOR'S PRESENTATION

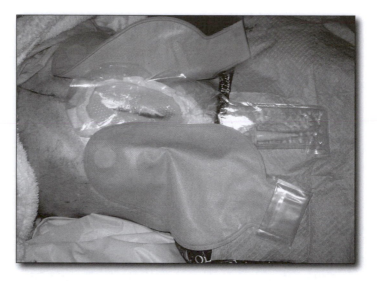

Figure 16.11 Fixation tape is used to reinforce security of the fistula appliance. This is applied to the edge and skin surface. The central fistula appliance is attached to a continuous drainage system at night to maximise rest and eliminate the need for frequent emptying.

AUTHOR'S PRESENTATION

Chapter 17

Lymphoedema

Avril Lunken

Introduction

Wounds do not result directly from the pathophysiology of lymphoedema, but any wounds that do occur are less likely to heal satisfactorily. Effective management of lymphoedema is therefore very important in managing wounds in persons with this condition.

This chapter considers lymphoedema and wound-care nursing under the following headings:

- anatomy and physiology of the lymph system;
- definition and classification of lymphoedema;
- signs and symptoms of lymphoedema;
- diagnosis of lymphoedema;
- lymphoedema and wound healing;
- complex decongestive therapy; and
- alternative treatments.

Anatomy and physiology of lymph system

The lymph system extends throughout the body at superficial and deeper levels. It includes such organs and tissues as the tonsils, spleen, thymus, lymph nodes, lymph vessels, and lymph fluid. The main functions of the lymph system are summarised in the Box below.

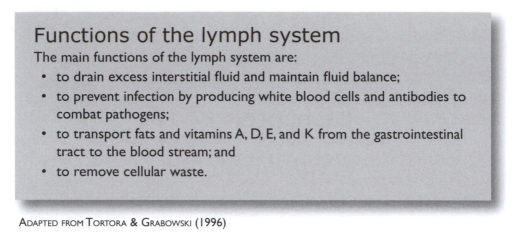

Functions of the lymph system

The main functions of the lymph system are:

- to drain excess interstitial fluid and maintain fluid balance;
- to prevent infection by producing white blood cells and antibodies to combat pathogens;
- to transport fats and vitamins A, D, E, and K from the gastrointestinal tract to the blood stream; and
- to remove cellular waste.

ADAPTED FROM TORTORA & GRABOWSKI (1996)

The functions of the lymph system summarised in the Box can be understood in terms of the functions of:

- lymph fluid;
- lymph vessels; and
- lymph nodes.
  Each of these is discussed below.

Lymph fluid

Lymph fluid contains water, protein, cells, cellular waste products, parasites, microorganisms, and various molecular structures.

The arterioles and capillaries move water, nutrients, and gases into tissues where cellular metabolism takes place. Once this process is complete, large molecular products pass through the lymph system for purification before being returned to the venous bloodstream. The lymph system pumps 2–4 litres of fluid per day (Tortora & Grabowski 1996). Lymph fluid is clear with a golden tinge; however, when it leaves the lower digestive tract, it often has a creamy-white appearance—due to lipid absorption.

Lymph fluid travels through lymph vessels and nodes to the lymph ducts. It is then returned to the venous blood system.

Lymph vessels

The transportation of lymph fluid begins in a multitude of tiny vessels known as *initial lymph capillaries*. These vessels have wide 'flap' entry points that allow entry of large protein molecules and cellular debris.

The fluid then moves into *lymph vessels*. These vessels have bands of muscle that pulsate at 5–7 beats per minute to keep the lymph moving (Weissleder & Schuchhardt 1997). Valves in the vessels ensure a one-way flow.

Deep in the body, the lymphatic vessels are larger, but fewer in number. The largest are known as *lymph ducts*. The main large vessel is known as the *thoracic duct*. It is 38–45 cm in length (Tortora & Grabowski 1996). The thoracic duct originates in the abdomen at the level of the second lumbar vertebra, and runs parallel with the spine until it joins the venous bloodstream at the subclavian junction (behind the left clavicle). It collects lymph from below the diaphragm and from the left side of

'The flow of lymph fluid is influenced by differential pressures and fluid concentrations ... and by other bodily activity.'

the body above the diaphragm. The *right lymphatic duct* collects lymph from the right side of the body above the diaphragm. This duct is only 1.25 cm in length. It begins at the base of the neck and joins the right subclavian vein behind the right clavicle.

The flow of lymph fluid is influenced by differential pressures and fluid concentrations in the arteries, veins, capillaries, interstitial fluid, and initial lymph vessels. Flow is also produced by other bodily activity—such as arterial pulsation, respiration, and ordinary body movement (such as walking, reaching, and bending).

Filtration, absorption, and reabsorption all occur during the passage of lymph fluid through the system.

Lymph nodes

Lymph nodes vary in size—from the size of a pinhead to that of a baked bean. The lymph nodes are 'strung together' along the lymph vessels—rather like a pearl necklace. The largest clusters of nodes occur in the neck, axilla, groin, and abdomen. Smaller clusters occur in the popliteal fossa (behind the knee) and cubital fossa (in front of the elbow). There are also many other nodes scattered throughout the body. It is estimated that there are 600–700 lymph nodes in the body (Weissleder & Schuchhardt 1997).

'Lymph nodes are vital for the body's defences ... filtering lymph fluid and destroying pathogens.'

Lymph nodes are vital for the body's defences. Reticular fibres within the nodes filter lymph fluid and destroy pathogens by producing lymphocytes and macrophages (white blood cells formed within the lymph system) and antibodies. For example, if a person with an infected throat has tender nodes under the mandible or in the neck, this indicates that the lymph system is working to protect the body.

Lymph nodes are sometimes incorrectly referred to as 'glands'.

Definition and classification of lymphoedema

Lymphoedema is an accumulation of excess fluid in the tissues caused by inadequate lymph drainage (BLS 2001). This accumulation of fluid, if left untreated, hinders normal cellular activity—ultimately leading to fibrotic and indurated tissue. It can affect any part of the body.

'Lymphoedema is an accumulation of excess fluid in the tissues caused by inadequate lymph drainage.'

Lymphoedema can be categorised as primary or secondary.

Primary lymphoedema occurs when the lymph system is incomplete, malformed, or nonexistent. The condition can be triggered at any time of life, and predominantly affects the lower limbs.

Secondary lymphoedema typically occurs as a result of trauma, radiotherapy, or surgery—particularly surgery that involves removal of lymph nodes. Scarring and lymph node removal create barriers to the usual pathways of lymph flow—thus causing fluid accumulation. People who have scarring as a result of one of the above events remain at life-long risk of developing lymphoedema. This can be triggered by seemingly

Classification of lymphoedema

Lymphoedema can be categorised as *primary* or *secondary*.

Primary lymphoedema

Primary lymphoedema occurs when the lymph system is incomplete, malformed, or nonexistent. The condition can be triggered at any time of life, and predominantly affects the lower limbs.

Secondary lymphoedema

Secondary lymphoedema occurs as a result of trauma, radiotherapy, or surgery. Scarring and lymph node removal create barriers to the usual pathways of lymph flow—thus causing fluid accumulation.

insignificant events, such as insect bites, scratches, sunburn, long car journeys, air travel, overuse of a limb, or infection.

Filariasis is a form of secondary lymphoedema induced by a tropical parasitic infection. The condition was previously known as 'elephantiasis'.

Obesity can have a negative effect on the lymph system. In both primary and secondary lymphoedema, obesity results in there being more tissue for the lymph to travel through.

Signs and symptoms of lymphoedema

People with lymphoedema describe various symptoms in the affected area. These include: feeling swollen, a 'bursting' sensation, tingling, tenderness, dull aching, tightness of the skin, a restricted range of movement, and temperature variations. Pain is unusual.

Signs of lymphoedema include swelling and pitting oedema. There might be a feeling of 'sponginess' in one limb as compared with the other.

If nurses detect the above signs and symptoms, referral to a doctor and a specialist lymphoedema therapist is indicated. An early diagnosis of lymphoedema enhances the patient's outcomes because the tissues are soft, treatment is comparatively simple, and changes to lifestyle are less problematic. If diagnosis is delayed, the situation is complicated on many levels. The tissues are likely to have become indurated, the risk of cellulitis will have increased, and treatment becomes more expensive. In addition, delayed diagnosis can have psychosocial consequences—including distorted body image, difficulties with intimate relationships, and the stigma associated with the bodily changes.

Diagnosis of lymphoedema

Differential diagnosis

Patients who do not have lymphoedema can present with signs and symptoms similar to those of lymphoedema. Because lymphoedema requires specific treatment, investigations to determine the correct diagnosis should be undertaken. Possible alternative diagnoses include:

- oedema;
- lipoedema; and
- myxoedema.

Oedema

Oedema is an abnormal accumulation of fluid in spite of a normally functioning lymph system. The condition often presents bilaterally and symmetrically.

Oedema can be caused by such conditions as heart disease, liver disease, renal disease, malnutrition (hypoalbuminaemia), vascular disorders, and immobility.

Oedema can coexist with lymphoedema. It is important to diagnose and treat the underlying condition before treating the lymphoedema (Piller & Eaton 2004).

Lipoedema

Lipoedema is a chronic disease with abnormal distribution of fatty tissue. The condition usually occurs bilaterally and symmetrically, and occurs more commonly in women. It rarely affects the upper limbs, feet, or hands. Signs and symptoms that can assist in diagnosing lipoedema include pain (even from light pressure) and easy bruising (Weissleder & Schuchhardt 1997).

Myxoedema

Myxoedema is associated with thyroid gland dysfunction leading to accumulation of mucoid fluid around the lower legs, eyes, lids, and hands (Weissleder & Schuchhardt 1997).

Diagnostic tools

A range of tools is available to assist with the diagnosis of lymphoedema. A thorough health and social history should be undertaken. This should be followed by examination using a tape measure or perometer to measure the limb. A perometer is a computerised measuring device that uses infrared rays to provide accurate length and circumference measurements of the limb. A tonometer and bio-impedance can be used to identify tissue changes.

More sophisticated investigations include magnetic resonance imaging (MRI), ultrasound, and lymphoscintigraphy (an isotope scan). These can be used for mapping the lymph system and lymph flow.

Lymphoedema and wound healing

Wounds do not result directly from the pathophysiology of lymphoedema, but any wounds that do occur are less likely to heal satisfactorily. Lymphoedema inhibits wound healing and decreases resistance to infection because the transport and activity of oxygen, nutrients, and white blood cells are diminished in the swollen areas. Effective lymphoedema management can reduce the swelling and improve the wound-healing process.

'Any wounds suffered by patients with lymphoedema should be treated immediately— even minor wounds.'

Any wounds suffered by patients with lymphoedema should be treated *immediately*—even minor wounds such as scratches, insect bites, or sunburn. This is especially important if these minor wounds occur in an area where the lymph system is compromised. Such areas are susceptible to infections, which can rapidly lead to cellulitis. Repeated episodes of cellulitis can further damage the lymph system.

If patients are referred with 'leg ulcers' or 'for treatment of oedema', nurses should be aware these people might have underlying lymphoedema—especially if wounds do not heal as expected. If there is uncertainty about the aetiology of the condition, nurses should refer the patient back to the doctor for further investigation.

Management of lymphoedema

Quality of life

The overriding goal of lymphoedema treatment is to improve quality of life for the patient. Nurses should be sensitive to the psychosocial issues involved with lymphoedema, and should provide lymphoedema education in its widest sense. This approach empowers patients to make choices that suit their life circumstances and enables them to manage their lymphoedema with the assistance of the therapist.

'The overriding goal of lymphoedema treatment is to improve quality of life for the patient.'

Nurses should be a source of encouragement, motivation, information, advice, and support for people with lymphoedema. Patients should be encouraged to experiment with the management of their condition, without fear of judgment or failure.

Complex decongestive therapy

Lymphoedema therapy is a specialist area of practice, and nurses and other health professionals should not undertake treatment of this condition without having received specialist training in the area.

The recommended treatment for lymphoedema is complex decongestive therapy (CDT). The components of CDT are:

- patient education;
- exercise;
- manual lymph drainage (MLD) treatment; and
- compression.

Each of these is discussed below.

Patient education

Patient education is fundamental to CDT. If patients have an understanding of their condition, compliance with treatment is enhanced. Education should include an explanation of the relevant anatomy and physiology, how lymphoedema develops, how it can be managed, and the long-term implications of the condition.

> *'Patient education is fundamental … If patients have an understanding of their condition, compliance with treatment is enhanced.'*

Advice should be given on diet, precautions, exercise, and skin care. In particular, patients should be advised that the risk of infection is decreased if the skin is kept moisturised and free from cracks and infection.

Complex decongestive therapy

This section of the text discusses complex decongestive therapy (CDT). The components of CDT discussed here are:

- patient education;
- exercise;
- manual lymph drainage (MLD) treatment; and
- compression.

Exercise

Exercise promotes lymph flow, strengthens muscles, and provides a sense of well-being. Patients should be advised to begin slowly, and then to increase exercise gently over a period of months. If the affected arm or leg develops heaviness, pain, or loss of power, the exercise program should be adjusted accordingly.

> *'Exercise promotes lymph flow, strengthens muscles, and provides a sense of well-being.'*

Abdominal breathing is a simple way to stimulate the whole lymph system. Changes in diaphragmatic pressure affect the flow of lymph upwards through the thoracic duct from its beginnings in the cisterna chyli in the abdomen.

When travelling, patients should be advised to avoid long periods of inactivity. Exercises for the ankle or the hand are recommended.

Manual lymph drainage

Manual lymph drainage (MLD) was first developed in Europe in the 1930s by Emil Vodder. Through a sequence of light, slow, rhythmical hand movements on the skin, MLD stimulates and redirects the lymph flow. Redirection removes excess lymph fluid from an area that has been compromised to an area that has not. Treatments are usually frequent and intensive—leading to a maintenance frequency once the swelling stabilises.

To alleviate symptoms, patients and family members can be taught a simplified version of MLD called 'simple lymph drainage' (SLD) (Bellhouse 2003).

MLD is different from traditional massages—in both objectives and technique. Nurses should not attempt MLD or SLD without specific training in its techniques.

Compression

Compression garments have a beneficial role in the management of lymphoedema. By applying a pressure gradient, compression garments assist the muscles in transporting lymph fluid upwards—thus preventing 'pooling'.

Compression garments can be knitted 'in the round' (like most hosiery) or tailored according to a patient's specific measurements. The compression in such garments is graded—100% at the ankle or wrist, approximately 75% at the knee or elbow, and 50% at the thigh or upper arm. The compression ranges from approximately 18.5 mm Hg to approximately 59 mm Hg.

Compression garments should be worn (and washed) every day to achieve the correct compression. They have a life expectancy of approximately 6 months (longer if looked after carefully and if two pairs are used alternately).

The garments are not easy to put on or remove. Manufacturers recommend the use of dishwashing gloves to ease the fabric along the limb. Gloves with serrations on the palms and fingers are best. Compression garment 'donners' are also available to assist with putting on garments.

Compression garments come in many styles, fabrics, weights, and colours. They can be purchased 'off the shelf' or 'made to measure'. Some clinics have subsidised schemes to defray patient costs in purchasing compression garments.

People with lymphoedema often fear the prospect of a lifetime of wearing such garments, but compromises can be made to allay these concerns—for example, wearing compression garments at particular 'risk times'—such as for air travel or heavy work.

'People often fear the prospect of a lifetime of wearing such garments, but compromises can be made to allay these concerns.'

It is sometimes necessary to use multi-layered compression bandaging to regain limb shape, reduce limb size, protect fragile skin, break down indurated tissue, and provide comfort. (See Chapter 11, 'Bandaging and Compression Therapy', page 171, for more on multi-layered compression therapy.) This treatment is usually offered on a daily basis for about two weeks in specialised clinics where the patient is monitored, measured, treated with MLD, and rebandaged. After two weeks, the aim is to fit single-layer compression garments because they are usually more comfortable, practicable, and easier for the patient to put on and take off.

A variety of aids is available to assist patients with exercise and the wearing of compression garments. Examples of these are:

- blow-up cushions or foam wedges—to facilitate small foot exercises;
- squeeze balls ('stress balls')—for exercising the forearm and hand; and
- 'donners'—fabric or metal frames to assist in putting on and removing compression garments.

Summary of CDT

All patients need to understand the concepts of CDT, and the purpose of each component. They are then able to incorporate this knowledge into their lifestyles, or at least know the risks if they do not.

Not everyone requires every component of CDT. The severity of lymphoedema determines the choice of components. Some patients might need to wear a compression garment only on certain occasions. Others might not be able to afford frequent regular MLD treatments—but it is desirable that such patients know how to self-massage. A process of trial and error is often required to ascertain which components of CDT are desirable for the quality of life of individual patients.

Alternative treatments

A number of other treatments exists for lymphoedema. Most have been developed and researched during the past two decades. When considering such treatments, patients should be advised to discuss them with a medical practitioner or a trained lymphoedema therapist. Examples of such treatments include:

- laser;
- surgery;
- compression pumps; and
- diuretics.

Laser

The application of low-level laser to affected limbs can significantly reduce lymphoedema (Carati et al. 2003). This treatment can be used in conjunction with CDT.

Surgery

Surgical 'debulking' has been used for many years to reduce gross lymphoedema. Other surgical procedures include microsurgical reconstruction (Baumeister et al. 1986) and specialist liposuction (Brorson et al. 1998).

Compression pumps

Compression pumps should be used only under the supervision of a lymphoedema therapist. The use of such pumps should be combined with components of CDT (especially MLD) (Board & Harlow 2002).

Diuretics

Diuretics are often used to treat lymphoedema, but they have only limited benefit. This is because they remove the fluid component of swelling, but leave behind cellular metabolic wastes. Over time, this can lead to fibrosis.

Conclusion

Lymphoedema is a chronic and life-changing condition. Although it cannot be cured, it can be managed successfully. In terms of wound-care nursing, lymphoedema is significant because it can impair wound healing.

Effective treatment consists of a number of techniques that have been discussed in this chapter—many of which require specialist training. However, in view of the significant psychosocial effects of the disease, the most significant aspect of wound-care treatment is the relationship that the nurse develops with the patient.

'The most significant aspect of wound-care treatment is the relationship that the nurse develops with the patient.'

Chapter 18

Dermatological Conditions

Genevieve Sadler and Michael Stacey

Introduction

Wound-care practitioners encounter a range of dermatological conditions, and multidisciplinary, individualised treatment is required to manage these conditions successfully. Nurses can assist in identifying and referring patients with dermatological conditions to appropriate medical practitioners.

The skin surrounding a wound is susceptible to certain problems, and many cutaneous diseases can present with ulceration. This chapter summarises the typical clinical features and management of some of the dermatological conditions associated with wounds. The framework of the chapter is shown in the Box on page 300.

Ulcerating dermatological conditions

This section describes some examples of ulcerating dermatological conditions. Most chronic wounds are due to venous insufficiency, arterial disease, diabetes, or pressure. These common conditions are described in detail elsewhere in this book. In contrast, the dermatological conditions

Framework of the chapter

This chapter discusses the clinical features and management of some of the dermatological conditions associated with wounds. The chapter is arranged as follows.

Ulcerating dermatological conditions
- Malignancies (page 301)
- Necrotising soft-tissue infections (page 302)
- Vasculitis (page 303)
- Calciphylaxis (page 305)
- Necrobiosis lipoidica diabeticorum (page 306)
- Martorell's ulcer (page 308)
- Pyoderma gangrenosum (page 308)

Peri-ulcer dermatological conditions
- Gravitational eczema (page 310)
- Allergic contact dermatitis (page 312)

Dermatological treatments
- Topical corticosteroids (page 313)
- Moisturisers (page 315)

described in this chapter are relatively rare. They should be considered if an ulcer has any of the following features:

- no evidence of common aetiologies;
- an atypical appearance; or
- no reduction in size after four weeks of appropriate treatment.

A thorough assessment of each patient is imperative. A skin biopsy at the ulcer edge is the most useful investigation. If there is any concern regarding unusual pathology, the patient should be referred for a second opinion.

It is important to be aware of the range of conditions that can cause ulceration. The correct treatment can be instigated only when the correct diagnosis is made. Dermatological conditions can be associated with serious underlying diseases, and can occasionally be life-threatening.

Malignancies

Approximately 4% of leg ulcers referred to specialised outpatient clinics are skin malignancies (Yang et al. 1996). The majority of these malignancies are basal cell carcinomas (BCCs), although squamous cell carcinomas (SCCs) and melanomas also ulcerate. In addition, longstanding ulceration of any cause can also undergo malignant change (known as a 'Marjolin's ulcer'). It is important to reassess wounds over time, regardless of the initial diagnosis.

Malignant ulcers typically have a raised appearance, an irregular base, and rolled borders. They often bleed easily. However, it can be impossible to distinguish a skin cancer from a non-malignant wound on examination. Malignancies are diagnosed on biopsy.

Excision is the treatment of choice for BCCs, SCCs, and melanomas. Left untreated, skin cancers cause increasing local tissue destruction. The risk of metastasis depends on the type of malignancy. BCCs rarely (if ever) metastasise, whereas 10% of melanomas have metastasised at the time of presentation.

'Patients who have had skin cancers are at risk of developing more skin cancers in the future.'

The patient's entire skin should be thoroughly examined to exclude coexisting skin cancers. Patients who have had skin cancers are at risk of developing more skin cancers in the future.

Ultraviolet radiation is the major cause of skin malignancies—and sun protection reduces the risk of future malignancies (Thompson, Jolley & Marks 1993). Patients should be advised to:

- limit sun exposure between 10 am and 3 pm;
- seek out the shade;
- wear a broad-brimmed hat;
- wear protective clothing; and
- use high-protection sun cream (SPF15 or higher).

Necrotising soft-tissue infections

Necrotising soft-tissue infections are characterised by extensive and rapid tissue damage. They are associated with significant morbidity and mortality.

Several specific syndromes have been described (DiNubile & Lipsky 2004):

- *necrotising fasciitis type 1*—due to mixed bacterial infection (including *Streptococcus pyogenes*, Gram-negative bacteria, and anaerobes);
- *necrotising fasciitis type 2*—due to *Streptococcus pyogenes*;
- *Fournier's gangrene*—necrotising fasciitis affecting the male perineum;
- *myonecrosis (gas gangrene)*—due to Clostridium species; and
- *progressive superficial synergistic gangrene*—due to microaerophilic streptococcus combined with either *Staphylococcus aureus* or Gram-negative bacteria.

Necrotising soft-tissue infections tend to occur in immunocompromised patients (especially persons with diabetes) and often follow surgery or trauma. The lower limb, abdomen, and perineum are the most commonly affected sites.

Typically, the wound consists of three zones: (i) a central area of necrosis; (ii) a surrounding violaceous (purplish) margin; and (iii) an outer bright erythematous zone. See Figure 18.1 (page 303).

The infection can spread through the subcutaneous tissues without major skin changes, and is sometimes misdiagnosed as cellulitis. Patients often report severe wound pain and are systemically unwell.

Necrotising soft-tissue infections are treated with extensive surgical debridement and broad-spectrum antibiotics. Early treatment is essential to minimise progression to septic shock and death.

Patients with necrotising fasciitis have a very poor prognosis. If nurses suspect that a patient might have signs of a necrotising soft-tissue infection, prompt referral to a medical practitioner is essential.

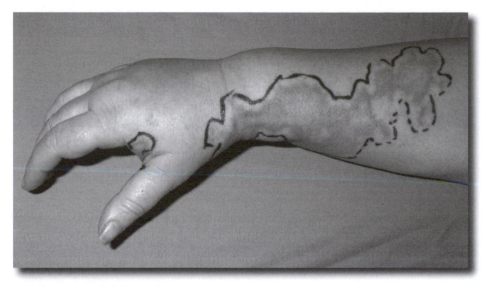

Figure 18.1 Necrotising fasciitis
AUTHORS' PRESENTATION

Vasculitis

Ulcers due to vasculitis are often mistaken for venous or arterial leg ulcers. However, vasculitis is the result of inflammation of blood vessel walls, not circulatory insufficiency.

The clinical picture depends on the size and site of the affected blood vessels. Cutaneous vasculitis can occur in isolation or can be associated with vasculitis in other organs. It can be idiopathic or secondary to other factors (for example, connective tissue diseases, infections, malignancies, or drugs).

Vasculitis can be classified into specific diseases. The diseases that are most relevant to wound-care practitioners are shown in Table 18.1, page 304.

Skin changes are most commonly seen in association with small-vessel vasculitis. These changes usually occur on the lower limb, but can occur anywhere on the body. Signs include:

- *palpable purpura*—raised, non-blanching, red lesions due to haemorrhage from affected blood vessels (see Figure 18.2, page 305);

- *subcutaneous nodules*—can be tender; due to inflammatory masses around affected blood vessels; and
- *ulceration*—typically painful with a necrotic base; due to obstruction or destruction of affected blood vessels.

Early in the course of vasculitis, patients often describe a 'flu-like' illness—with fever, malaise, and arthralgia.

Table 18.1 Vasculitis conditions relevant to wound care
AUTHORS' PRESENTATION (ADAPTED FROM CHARLES & FALK 1997)

Disease	Vessel involved	Clinical features	Pathological features
Polyarteritis nodosa	Small–medium	Ischaemia in affected organs (for example, lower limb claudication and ulceration) Subcutaneous nodules	Arterial stenosis due to active inflammation or subsequent scarring
Wegener's granulomatosis	Small–medium	Sinus pain; discharge; fistula Lung infiltrates Nephritis	Usually positive serum antineutrophil cytoplasmic antibody (ANCA)
Henoch-Schonlein purpura	Small	Palpable purpura Gastrointestinal bleeding Nephritis Arthritis	Immunoglobulin A dominant immune complex deposition Often follows an upper respiratory tract infection
Cryoglobulinaemic vasculitis	Small	Palpable purpura Ulceration Nephritis Arthritis	Cryoglobulin deposition Often associated with Hepatitis C
Cutaneous leukocytoclastic vasculitis	Small	Palpable purpura Ulceration	Idiopathic or associated with connective tissue diseases, infections, malignancies, or drugs

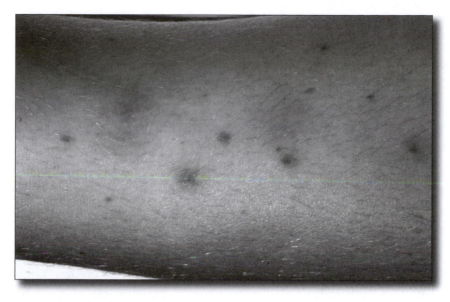

Figure 18.2 Palpable purpura
AUTHORS' PRESENTATION

The diagnosis of cutaneous vasculitis requires a skin biopsy and blood tests for inflammatory markers and autoantibodies. Investigations should also be undertaken to detect whether there is involvement of other organs and any underlying diseases. It can be difficult to establish a specific diagnosis, and many specialists might have to be involved.

Treatment varies according to the type of vasculitis. It often involves immunosuppressants—such as steroids or cyclophosphamide. Underlying conditions must be treated.

The outlook for these patients is variable. A patient with drug-induced leukocytoclastic vasculitis is unlikely to experience recurrent problems once the offending drug has been ceased. In contrast, patients with Wegener's granulomatosis tend to have a remitting and relapsing course, and are at risk of developing significant renal impairment.

Calciphylaxis

Calciphylaxis is also known as calcific uraemic arteriolopathy. It is characterised by progressive calcification of the cutaneous vasculature, and is usually associated with end-stage renal disease (ESRD) and hyperparathyroidism. However, only 1% of patients with ESRD develop this complication each year (Budisavljevic, Cheek & Ploth 1996).

The aetiology of calciphylaxis is unknown. Calcium is deposited in the walls of small and medium-sized subcutaneous blood vessels. This leads to vessel obstruction, inflammation in the surrounding fat, and necrosis of overlying skin.

Typical lesions commence as violaceous nodules or plaques on the abdomen or lower limb. These progress to necrotic ulcers, covered with an eschar. Calciphylaxis occurs suddenly and evolves rapidly. Patients often report severe ulcer pain.

The diagnosis requires biopsy of the ulcer. Distinctive histopathology allows the clinical diagnosis to be confirmed. However, the clinician should have a high index of suspicion for co-existing obstruction of the large arteries.

The management of calciphylaxis is controversial. Patients can benefit from parathyroidectomy or phosphate-binding medication. It is also advisable to avoid potential triggers—such as trauma and immunosuppression. However, the outlook for these patients remains poor—with a mortality rate of up to 80% due to wound infection and progressive renal failure (Ledbetter, Khoshnevis & Hsu 2000).

An example of a patient with calciphylaxis and peripheral arterial disease is presented in the Box on page 307. The story of Mr D illustrates that there can be more than one cause for cutaneous ulceration.

Necrobiosis lipoidica diabeticorum

Necrobiosis lipoidica diabeticorum (NLD) is a skin lesion that is characteristically associated with diabetes mellitus (Margolis 1995), although it can occasionally occur in patients before the onset of diabetes or in those who never develop diabetes. It is most commonly seen in young females.

Classic NLD lesions are atrophic, orange-yellow plaques over the pre-tibial region. Ulceration, which occurs in less than 30% of these lesions, is typically superficial. However, biopsy has demonstrated that

More than one cause for ulceration

Mr D was a 65-year-old man with end-stage renal failure and hypercalcaemia. He developed painful ulceration of his right gaiter region. The ulcer and surrounding skin was necrotic (see Figure 18.3, below).

Biopsy confirmed calciphylaxis. A parathyroidectomy was performed, and Mr D's serum calcium returned to normal. However, the ulcers did not improve and a new ulcer developed on the right great toe. Pedal pulses were noted to be weak bilaterally.

An angiogram showed left femoral artery stenosis and a bypass procedure was performed. The pain improved dramatically and the ulcer healed two-months later.

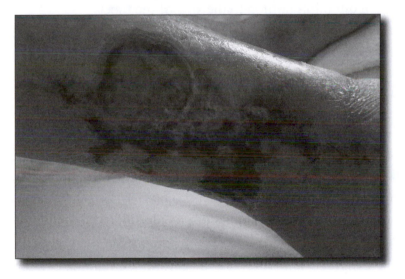

Figure 18.3 Calciphylaxis
AUTHORS' PRESENTATION

the process is more extensive, with diffuse collagen destruction and inflammation through the lower dermis.

Treatment of NLD is usually unsuccessful. The most promising treatment is antiplatelet medication (aspirin and dipyridamole)

(Margolis 1995). Other treatments that can be tried include topical or oral steroids, hyperbaric oxygen, pentoxifylline, and nicotinamide.

Good diabetic control is undoubtedly important for the patient's general health, but its benefit for the ulcerating skin lesions is controversial.

Martorell's ulcer

Martorell's ulcer is a syndrome of painful lower limb ulceration usually associated with severe, prolonged hypertension.

The typical patient with a Martorell's ulcer is a female aged between 50 and 70 years (Shutler, Baragwanath & Harding 1995). Lesions usually occur on the outside of the lower limb, and can be symmetrical. Purpuric areas rapidly ulcerate, showing a necrotic base. Ulcer pain is significant, and can seem out of proportion to the size of the ulcer.

Ulcer biopsy is not diagnostic. The changes seen in Martorell's ulcers are identical to those seen in the skin of hypertensive patients without ulceration. It is essential to exclude vasculitis and large vessel obstruction before making a diagnosis of Martorell's ulcer.

Treatment involves control of any underlying hypertension. Beta-blocker medications should be avoided because they cause peripheral vasoconstriction and can impair wound healing (Mekkes et al. 2003).

Martorell's ulcers usually heal in 4–12 months. However recurrence occurs in up to 80% of patients.

Pyoderma gangrenosum

Pyoderma gangrenosum (PG) is a chronic inflammatory condition characterised by neutrophil infiltration of the dermis. The pathogenesis is poorly understood but is likely to involve an abnormal immune response. More than half of affected patients suffer from other medical conditions—such as inflammatory bowel disease, rheumatoid arthritis, or haematological malignancies (Callen 1998).

Patients typically present with a painful nodule or pustule that rapidly evolves into an ulcer with undermined violaceous borders. Lesions most commonly develop on the lower limb.

Biopsy can be used to support a clinical diagnosis of PG, but this is not diagnostic. Specialist review is required to exclude other conditions that mimic PG (Weening, Davis & Dahl 2002). In particular, underlying infection should be ruled out before immunosuppressant therapy is commenced.

A variety of treatments has been suggested (Chow & Ho 1996). Management can include:

- treatment of underlying condition and any associated diseases;
- local therapy—such as topical sodium cromoglycate, tacrolimus, or intralesional steroids (for early or mild lesions);
- systemic therapy—such as steroids or cyclosporine (for more severe cases); and
- avoidance of aggressive debridement—because these lesions can be exacerbated by trauma (see Box, below).

Pyoderma gangrenosum exacerbated by trauma

Mrs E was a 55-year-old woman with rheumatoid arthritis. A painful, rapidly enlarging ulcer developed from a pustule on her right gaiter region. The ulcer is shown in Figure 18.4 (page 310). It had a sloughy base, bright red-blue wound edges, and surrounding erythema.

A wound infection was diagnosed and Mrs E was admitted to hospital for intravenous antibiotics. The ulcer did not improve, so it was debrided. After surgery, the ulcer rapidly increased in size.

Biopsy was consistent with pyoderma gangrenosum, and there was no underlying infection. High dose intravenous steroids were commenced. The pain decreased and the ulcer began to heal.

This case illustrates how this condition can be exacerbated by debridement or other trauma.

No therapeutic agent is uniformly effective. In practice, a variety of agents might be trialled over time to determine which is best.

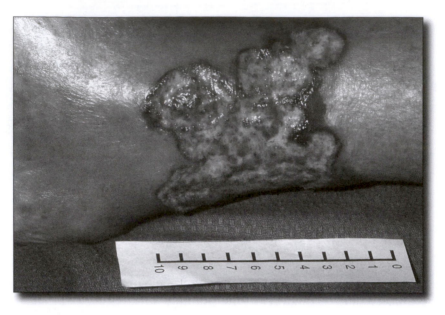

Figure 18.4 Pyoderma gangrenosum
AUTHORS' PRESENTATION

Pyoderma gangrenosum has an unpredictable course (Von den Dreisch 1997). Most cases improve initially, but ongoing treatment is required to prevent recurrence.

Peri-ulcer dermatological conditions

Gravitational eczema

Gravitational eczema (also known as stasis dermatitis, venous eczema, or varicose eczema) is an inflammatory eruption of the lower limbs due to venous hypertension. It occurs in more than one-third of patients with venous leg ulceration, and can also occur without ulceration (Patel, Llewellyn & Harding 2001). This condition often makes patients scratch—thereby impairing healing or precipitating new wounds.

Gravitational eczema is diagnosed on clinical grounds. Signs include:

- diffuse erythema;
- dryness;

- scaling;
- weeping; and
- excoriations.

Eczema is typically seen in the gaiter region, but can extend from the knees to the feet.

Treatment of gravitational eczema involves a combination of therapies (Patel, Llewellyn & Harding 2001):

- treatment of venous hypertension—usually with compression bandages (or bed rest and leg elevation for severe cases);
- avoidance of irritants—which commonly include heat, cold, excessive moisture, and wool;
- moisturisers—aiming to reduce dryness and scaling;
- astringents—such as potassium permanganate (to reduce weeping);
- paste bandages—which can be soothing and protect the skin from scratching;
- oral antibiotics—cellulitis frequently complicates eczema because excoriated areas provide a portal of entry for infection; and
- topical steroids.

It is important to be aware of all topical therapies used by the patient so that he or she can be advised to discontinue potentially harmful self-therapies (such as household antiseptics).

'If a topical steroid appears ineffective, the common response is to increase the potency ... A more appropriate response might be to provide help with the application of the original medication.'

The patient's ability to apply topical preparations needs to be explored. If a topical steroid appears ineffective, the common response is to increase the potency of the preparation. A more appropriate response might be to provide help with the application of the original medication.

These patients typically experience recurrent flares and remissions of symptoms.

Once an episode of gravitational eczema has resolved, measures can be implemented to reduce the risk of recurrence. These include ongoing compression therapy, avoidance of irritants, and frequent use of moisturisers.

Allergic contact dermatitis

Allergic contact dermatitis is an inflammatory skin eruption in response to exposure to an allergen. This is very common in patients with venous leg ulcers, with up to 75% of patients becoming sensitised to specific allergens (compared with 2% of the general population who develop allergies) (Machet et al. 1994).

Allergic contact dermatitis can have a similar appearance to gravitational eczema on clinical examination. However, suspicion of allergic contact dermatitis should be raised if:

- the eczema persists despite intensive treatment for gravitational eczema; or
- the eczema is localised to the area of a dressing or topical therapy, and is sharply demarcated.

'The most important aspect of management is to avoid the identified allergens.'

The reaction can also occur in skin that has not had direct contact with the allergen.

An example of allergic contact dermatitis is illustrated in Figure 18.5, page 313.

Diagnosis requires patch testing. In this procedure, patches of potential allergens are applied to the patient's back for 2–3 days. The skin reactions are measured on removal, and again after a further two days.

Potential allergens include lanolin (present in many moisturisers), rubber (present in certain bandages and latex gloves), corticosteroids (especially hydrocortisone), and mupirocin (a topical antibiotic).

The most important aspect of management is to avoid the identified allergens. Acute episodes require potent topical steroids, astringents, and moisturisers. Nurses should be aware of the composition of products that they are applying to patients or that patients are using for self-treatment. If the nurse and patient work together, potential allergens can be identified and eliminated from the treatment regimen.

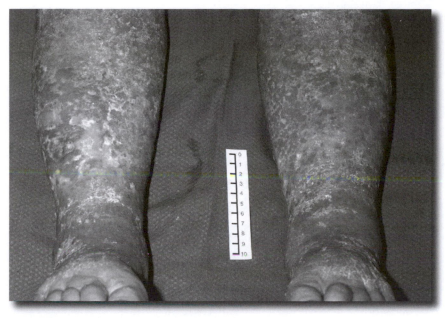

Figure 18.5 Allergic contact dermatitis
AUTHORS' PRESENTATION

Dermatological treatments

Topical corticosteroids

Topical corticosteroids are the most common form of treatment used by dermatologists. This group of medications can be both beneficial and harmful. Their use must be tailored to the patient, the dermatological condition, and the affected body site. General advice on topical corticosteroids is summarised in the Box on page 314.

Many patients are concerned about the risk of side-effects of topical corticosteroids.

Local side-effects include:

- skin atrophy;
- folliculitis;
- pigment disturbance;
- telangiectasia; and
- steroid allergy.

Use of topical corticosteroids

The following hints should be kept in mind when using topical corticosteroids.

Indications

- Use topical steroids only if a steroid-responsive condition has been diagnosed.
- Apply corticosteroids until the skin has become normal, and then cease.

Titration and strength

- Titrate potency of steroid to the severity of the condition (see Table 18.2, page 315).
- Mild disease flares can be treated with mild steroids. If there is no response after use of mild steroids for a few days, use a more potent steroid.
- Apply only mild steroids to areas with thin skin—such as the face.

Ointments and creams

- Use ointment if affected skin is dry, or if allergic contact dermatitis is a concern.
- Use cream if affected skin is weeping or folliculitis is a concern.

Frequency and dose

- Most steroids need to be applied only once per day.
- To measure the amount of steroid, one 'fingertip unit' contains 0.5 gram of ointment (which is enough to cover two palm areas of skin).

Occlusive dressings

- Covering the skin with occlusive or wet dressings after steroid application increases the absorption up to 100 times.
- This can be used for a few days in particularly severe flare-ups of a condition.

ADAPTED FROM LEE & MARKS (1998)

Table 18.2 Examples of topical steroids

AUTHORS' PRESENTATION (ADAPTED FROM LEE & MARKS 1998)

Class 1 (mild)	Class 2 (moderate)	Class 3 (potent)	Class 4 (very potent)
Hydrocortisone 0.5–1%	Betamethasone valerate 0.02–0.05%	Mometasone furoate 0.1%	Halcinonide 0.1%
	Triamcinolone acetonide 0.02–0.05%	Betamethasone valerate 0.1%	Betamethasone valerate 0.05% in optimised vehicle
		Betamethasone diproprionate 0.05%	

Systemic side-effects include:

- suppression of hypothalamic–pituitary axis;
- diabetes mellitus;
- hypertension;
- peptic ulceration; and
- cataracts.

Although it is important to watch for these side-effects, patients can be reassured that side-effects are unlikely to occur if steroids are used appropriately.

Patients can also be disillusioned if their disease recurs after steroids are ceased—and some might say that steroids 'don't work'. It is often necessary to educate patients that *'Side-effects are unlikely to occur if steroids are used appropriately.'* topical steroids control symptoms, but do not cure the disease. Steroids might need to be restarted if the problem flares up again. However, having a short break from steroids is useful in preventing a reduction in drug effect with prolonged treatment.

Moisturisers

Dry skin causes uncomfortable itching and exacerbates many dermatological conditions—such as gravitational eczema. Frequent use of moisturisers should be encouraged, especially in the elderly.

Examples of moisturisers include sorbolene, urea 10%, and white soft paraffin.

Their effectiveness can be maximised by:

- applying immediately after bathing (which is when the skin absorbs best);
- frequent use (up to three times per day in severe eczema);
- ongoing use (even when eczema has resolved because this helps to prevent further exacerbations);
- avoiding factors that dry the skin (such as long or hot showers); and
- using a soap substitute.

Conclusion

When managing a patient with a chronic wound, common aetiologies (such as venous disease, arterial insufficiency, diabetes, and pressure) should be considered first. If the wound appears unusual, or if it is not responding to treatment, less common dermatological conditions should be considered. These diseases are often associated with serious systemic disease and can be life-threatening. Specific treatment is important in minimising patient morbidity and mortality, as well as healing the wound.

'Dermatological conditions are often associated with serious systemic disease and can be life-threatening.'

The skin surrounding the wound often demands attention. Common problems in patients with venous leg ulcers are gravitational eczema and allergic contact dermatitis. It is important to work closely with the patient in managing these problems.

Patients might ask nurses for advice regarding topical corticosteroids. Sometimes nurses are asked to help with the application of these preparations. By following some general guidelines, topical steroids can be used effectively, and side-effects can be minimised. Ongoing use of moisturisers is beneficial in many situations.

Chapter 19

Best Practice

Taliesin Ellis

Introduction

A simple definition of 'best practice' is practice that is based solely on the best available, research-based evidence. However, such a definition is limited because it does not take into account individual clinical expertise and individual patient circumstances. What is 'best practice' in one set of circumstances might not be best practice in another set of circumstances. Nurses therefore require a range of options in the management of people with wounds. 'Best practice' for one patient might not be 'best practice' for another—even if their wounds are similar (Sackett et al. 1996; Guyatt, Cook & Haynes 2004; Reilly 2004).

If such an individualised approach were taken to an extreme, it would lead to 'best practice' being defined in terms of what works best for an individual—rather than in terms of a single practice approach. However, this sort of individualised definition would not provide any general guidance for practice.

The most useful working definition of 'best practice' is therefore gained by combining a generalised approach *and* an individualised approach. Best practice can then be defined as practice that accounts for the needs of the individual, recognises clinical expertise, and incorporates the best available research-based evidence.

Framework of the chapter

This chapter discusses best practice in wound care under the following headings:

- Evidence-based health care (page 318)
- Evidence in wound management (page 319)
- Quantitative research (page 320)—Ranking evidence (page 320); Systematic reviews (page 322); Meta-analyses (page 323)
- Qualitative research (page 323)
- Non-research based evidence: expert opinion (page 324)
- Determining best practice (page 325)
- Standards and clinical practice guidelines (page 328)
- Policies and procedures (page 330)

Evidence-based health care

Evidence-based health care (EBHC) has become the dominant paradigm in health care—both within the literature and in the practice community (Sackett et al. 1996; Forbes & Griffiths 2002; Parker 2002; Guyatt, Cook & Haynes 2004; Reilly 2004; Straus & Jones 2004). According to this dominant EBHC paradigm, best practice in wound management has thus come to be judged on the basis of the *evidence that underpins practice*—not merely on outcomes. Indeed, the term 'best practice' has become so synonymous with EBHC that the two are often used interchangeably—as if one implies the other (NHMRC 2000a, 2000b). Best practice must therefore incorporate the best available evidence, and it must be subject to change when new or better evidence becomes available.

'Evidence-based health care has become the dominant paradigm in health care.'

In EBHC, best practice is often defined by clinical practice guidelines (CPGs). These are, in effect, guides to the delivery of EBHC in a practice setting. CPGs are statements that have been formulated by consensus among experts in their fields who have analysed research-based evidence and considered expert opinion on clinical experience (NHMRC 2000a, 2000b). By consulting appropriate CPGs, practitioners can thus avail themselves of a combination of the best available evidence and experience to provide the best possible treatment options—in other words, EBHC (Sackett et al. 1996; NHMRC 2000a, 2000b; Guyatt, Cook & Haynes 2004).

'Wound management is varied and dynamic, and practice in this field is constantly under review.'

The notion that best practice incorporates both research-based evidence *and* a consensus on validated experience is especially important in wound management. Wound management is varied and dynamic, and practice in this field is constantly under review.

Evidence in wound management

In ancient times, collective wisdom on treatment of wounds was passed from generation to generation by word of mouth, and was eventually recorded in written form (Bibbings 1984; Carville 1993). This collective wisdom was the sum total of people's experience and was refined over time according to *outcomes*. However, during the past 200 years, evidence has begun to take on a different connotation under the influence of Western medicine (Sackett et al. 1996), and there is now an expectation that practice will be governed by evidence formulated through methodologically sound, replicable research—rather than by hearsay or experience (Parker 2000).

'There is now an expectation that practice will be governed by evidence formulated through research—rather than by hearsay or experience.'

There is a vast body of evidence related to the science of *healing*. However, in *wound management*, the research methods and measurements of outcomes can vary widely. In wound management, *blinded* randomised controlled trials (blinded RCTs) are difficult to implement because it is difficult to conceal any given practice variation being studied.

For example, it is difficult to 'conceal' the use of a hydrocolloid dressing as opposed to the use of saline soaks. In addition, it is difficult to control for all human physical, psychological, and social variables.

Apart from these problems, many wound-management products make their way onto the market once *safety* is established, but without significant studies having been performed on *efficacy*. Sometimes the practitioner's experience is the only 'evidence' that exists—and this type of 'evidence' is open to criticism under the EBHC practice model. Nurses should therefore recognise the limitations of research evidence in wound management and appreciate the need to evaluate wound-management research on its merits before deciding to base their practice upon it.

> *'Sometimes the practitioner's experience is the only "evidence" that exists.'*

Quantitative research

Ranking evidence

In EBHC, the best evidence is usually considered to be significant research-based outcomes derived from quantitative studies (Forbes & Griffiths 2002; Winch, Creedy & Chaboyer 2002; Guyatt, Cook & Haynes 2004), and various reputable bodies have devised ranking systems for research-based evidence. These bodies include the Cochrane Collaboration (UK), the National Health and Medical Research Council (Australia), the National Institute for Clinical Excellence (UK), and the Institute of Medicine (USA).

> *'The best evidence is usually considered to be significant research-based outcomes derived from quantitative studies.'*

Research results obtained from systematic reviews (SRs) of double-blinded RCTs are considered the 'gold standard' for research-based evidence. Ranked below this gold standard are results from other types of research designs. The lowest-ranked evidence consists of case series. Table 19.1, page 321 shows a suggested ranking of levels of evidence (NHMRC 1999).

Table 19.1 Levels of evidence

Author's presentation adapted from NHMRC (1999)

Level of evidence	Study design
1	Evidence obtained from a systematic review of all relevant randomised controlled trials
2	Evidence obtained from at least one properly designed randomised controlled trial
3.1	Evidence obtained from well-designed pseudo-randomised controlled trials (alternate allocation or some other method)
3.2	Evidence obtained from comparative studies (including systematic reviews of such studies) with concurrent controls and allocation not randomised, cohort studies, case-control studies, or interrupted time series with a control group
3.3	Evidence obtained from comparative studies with historical control, two or more single arm studies, or interrupted time series without a parallel control group
4	Evidence obtained from case series—either post-test, or pre-test and post-test

It should be noted that there are many ranking systems to rate the strength of evidence underpinning the efficacy of a particular practice or intervention. However, the various bodies that produce evidence-ranking systems recognise that single measures are not enough to rank evidence, and all recommend that summaries of evidence should be presented to broaden the scope of any piece of evidence and to be more inclusive. These summaries provide a better context for the interpretation of results, and are especially useful if 'gold-standard' levels of evidence do not exist.

When CPGs are produced, each practice guideline or set of recommendations is associated with an evidence rating so that the user is able to discern its relative strength or weakness. Treatment choices that are made in light of an evidence ranking are better informed, and expectations can be adjusted accordingly. Education can also be conducted to inform the patient of the merits of an intervention, and this can contribute to improved expectations and decision making.

Because there is such a variety of evidence-ranking systems, nurses should be aware of the ranking system used in each case to ensure that accurate, informed decisions are made.

Systematic reviews

Systematic reviews (SRs) are used to locate, appraise, and synthesise research results (NHMRC 2000a, 2000b; Forbes & Griffiths 2002; Traynor 2002; Winch, Creedy & Chaboyer 2002). An SR is a criterion-based process that organises and ranks results into a cohesive report informing a particular research or practice question.

'A systematic review is a criterion-based process that organises and ranks results into a cohesive report.'

A researcher conducting an SR on a particular intervention utilises a review protocol that includes or excludes certain levels of evidence and studies of a particular quality. The researcher can then report on the strength of evidence that exists—according to the protocol applied. This evidence can be used to determine best practice in respect of that particular intervention—that is, to develop relevant guidelines for practice, based on the evidence available.

An example of a wound-management research question might be: 'What is the evidence supporting the use of low air-loss mattresses in the treatment of stage 2 pressure ulcers?'. The outcome of an SR of this question might be a report suggesting that there are positive healing outcomes associated with the use of such mattresses compared with not using them.

'A systematic review is a key method for determining and articulating best practice.'

The strength of evidence might be rated as '2' (as per Table 19.1, page 321)—showing that there is sound support for this intervention. In this way, the SR can be used to determine that best practice for treatment of stage 2 pressure ulceration would incorporate the use of low air-loss mattresses. An SR is thus a key method for determining and articulating best practice in the EBHC paradigm.

Meta-analyses

If several studies have used the same quantitative research method, the outcomes from all of these studies can be combined and grouped. The 'grouping' of the results of such similar studies in this way is called 'meta-analysis'.

'Meta-analysis increases the significance and power of results.'

Meta-analysis increases the significance and power of results (Droogan & Song 1996; Greener & Grimshaw 1996; Forbes & Griffiths 2002; Kitson 2002). It is used to demonstrate the power of results that have been analysed or to highlight inconsistencies in results—thereby providing better information about the efficacy of a given intervention (Droogan & Song 1996; Greener & Grimshaw 1996; Forbes & Griffiths 2002; Kitson 2002).

If a meta-analysis can be performed, it is one of the strongest features of an SR. For this reason, SRs tend to sit atop the evidence rankings. Best practice is thus commonly considered to be practice that is based on guidelines which utilise findings from SRs that contain meta-analysis (Johnson 1988; Droogan & Song 1996; Greener & Grimshaw 1996; NHMRC 2000a, 2000b; Forbes & Griffiths 2002; Kitson 2002).

Qualitative research

Qualitative research is largely characterised by description, rather than by prediction (Reed & Procter 1995). It tends to focus on the 'why' rather than the 'what', and has contextual attributes.

'Qualitative research is largely characterised by description, rather than by prediction.'

Qualitative research methodology is commonly used in the social sphere, but it also has relevance in physiological research if there is a definite relationship between the psychosocial and physiological aspects of a subject. Because living with a wound involves both physiological *and* social factors, much of wound management can be studied with qualitative research methods.

Qualitative research helps practitioners to understand the *experiences* of people—for example, pain, comfort, happiness, satisfaction, effort, and motivation (Reed & Procter 1995). Collecting data on such experiences assists practice by adding depth and scope to the decisions faced by practitioners. Rather than making a decision that is based purely on physical efficacy (that is, what works best at the physical level), a practitioner can make decisions that take into account how a person might *experience* the treatment.

By using qualitative descriptive data, practice is better informed and more context-specific. Qualitative data should therefore be considered as valid evidence—despite the inherent subjectivity of such data. However, the use of qualitative data as evidence is not without problems. The subjective nature of data collected by qualitative studies leads to these studies having a lower ranking on the 'levels-of-evidence' scales used in the conduct of traditional SRs (Forbes & Griffiths 2002). Because these studies are often conducted with small, specifically chosen populations, there are difficulties in generalising from such studies. In addition, because populations are not always randomised or specifically controlled, the data can contain bias that is not properly accounted for.

'The quality and rigour of qualitative studies must be carefully assessed to ensure that bias or lack of generalisability does not affect outcomes.'

For these reasons, the quality and rigour of qualitative studies must be carefully assessed to ensure that bias or lack of generalisability does not affect outcomes. It *is* necessary to accept the context-specific nature of qualitative data, but this does *not* imply that data of poor quality should be accepted. If guidelines were to be generated from such data, this could lead to negative patient outcomes.

It is vital to assess the quality of *all* studies—whether the study is quantitative or qualitative. The validity of data is dependent on the strength and application of the study method, and the data generated must be assessed in light of the overall quality of the research.

Non-research based evidence: expert opinion

Historically, the collective experience of 'experts' has been highly respected. The advent of EBHC has decreased the weight given to expert opinion—but expert opinion should not be entirely discounted. To omit expert opinion *when there is no research-based evidence* would create a practice vacuum (NHMRC 2000a, 2000b).

If expert opinion is the only basis for practice, it should be a *starting-point* for further investigation—rather than being an end-point in itself. By recognising expert opinion in the formulation of guidelines, a practice trend or direction is created, and research-based evidence (as it becomes available) can then be used to validate or modify the opinion.

'Expert opinion … should be a starting-point for further investigation—rather than an end-point in itself.'

Expert opinion has sometimes been the *only* basis for judging 'best practice'. In these circumstances it has acquired the status of 'evidence' for best practice. However, issues such as bias, ego, and loyalty have meant that expert opinion is now given a low ranking (or not included at all) on evidence 'scales'. Expert opinion should therefore not be regarded as evidence *per se*, and if a practice recommendation is based on such expert opinion, the origin of that recommendation should be made clear (NHMRC 2000a, 2000b). In this way appropriate recognition is afforded to expert opinion, but without giving it the same status as research-based evidence.

'Appropriate recognition is afforded to expert opinion, but without giving it the same status as research-based evidence.'

Determining best practice

The hierarchy of evidence that is employed in an SR can, in itself, be quite limiting. The 'evidence hierarchy' reduces the relevance of any findings that have not been not elicited in the manner of an RCT. If findings other than RCTs are ignored, directional shifts in practice that are based on 'lower' levels of evidence are not included in reviews. This reduces opportunities to debate practice issues. It can even place certain practice areas outside the realm of EBHC.

This, in turn, can influence the directions given in CPCs and can thus reduce their applicability. For example, if there is no 'gold-standard' evidence to support a given practice, there is a chance that a potentially efficacious practice might be abandoned or ignored (Kitson 2002; Traynor 2002; Winch, Creedy & Saboyer 2002; Guyatt, Cook & Haynes 2004; Reilly 2004). And if a principle of practice is supported only by expert opinion, it might be concluded that the evidence is too weak to be considered, and that the principle is therefore unfounded. This can lead to directionless practice. In contrast, a more useful outcome might be achieved by placing the principle 'on notice'—and fostering more specific investigation of it.

Much of wound-management practice does not lend itself to examination by RCTs. This can mean that an SR of data collected about a particular wound-management intervention might find 'no evidence' (from RCTs) about that intervention—thus bringing the intervention into question. However, other data about that intervention might exist—rigorously derived from a method different from an RCT. Excluding such data from an SR synthesis can lead to limited practice options, and limited scope within CPCs. This reliance on only published research data is a problem with the SR method.

'Much of wound-management practice does not lend itself to examination by randomised, controlled studies.'

In addition, there can be bias within SR findings. Possible sources of bias within data collected for an SR include: (i) a tendency not to publish findings that are considered 'negative'; (ii) selective presentation of data; and (iii) prejudice in favour of the intervention being tested (Forbes & Griffiths 2002). These problems mean that an SR cannot be considered absolutely reliable. Practices that appear to be 'best practice' might have negative consequences that are unreported or unforeseen.

Best practice is therefore most accurately described as practice based on the 'best available' evidence. This evidence includes:

- systematic reviews and meta-analyses;
- published and unpublished data derived from high-quality quantitative and qualitative studies; and
- case studies representing clinical expertise and valid experience.

SRs are thus an effective method of determining the quality of data (and thereby assessing the outcomes of particular interventions), but they are not without their weaknesses and practitioners should therefore use them with a recognition of their limitations.

'Practitioners should use systematic reviews with a recognition of their limitations.'

Expert opinion should not be treated as 'evidence', but if other evidence does not exist, it can be used to guide practice. Useable expert opinion is often found in books, journal articles, and on the Internet, but practitioners should ensure that these sources of 'expert opinion' are contemporary, referenced, and peer-reviewed.

Case studies published in peer-reviewed journals can drive practice directions, but they should be viewed with caution because results tend to be patient-specific—that is, they cannot always be generalised.

'Best practice can be derived from the best available evidence—allowing for practice that is adaptable to situations and individuals.'

In summary, 'best practice' can be derived from principles formulated upon the best available evidence—allowing for practice that is adaptable to situations and individuals. This is especially important in wound management.

Summary of best practice in wound management

Best practice in wound management is most accurately described as practice based on the 'best available' evidence. This evidence includes:

- systematic reviews and meta-analyses;
- published and unpublished data derived from high-quality quantitative and qualitative studies; and
- case studies representing clinical expertise and valid experience.

Standards and clinical practice guidelines

Standards

Standards represent the 'ideal' in terms of expected treatment. They are benchmarks against which the application of healthcare processes can be measured. The expectation is that best practice should be consistent with the stated standards.

'Best practice is not always measured against outcomes based on research alone; rather, it should reflect the needs and desires of the patient.'

Standards are not always based on research-based evidence. Rather, standards often take into account professional, social, and individual ideals or needs. In this way, standards define best practice for individuals *in given circumstances*. Best practice is not always measured against outcomes based on research alone; rather, it should reflect the needs and desires of the patient.

Most national or international wound-management organisations (such as the Australian Wound Management Association and the World Union of Wound Healing Societies) have published documents that represent appropriate standards of care.

'It is in the interests of practitioners and patients alike that standards are applied within care plans, care approaches, and interventions.'

Standards are increasingly being used to determine whether best practice has been carried out, and it is in the interests of practitioners and patients alike that standards are applied within care plans, care approaches, and interventions.

Clinical practice guidelines

CPGs are different from standards of care. CPGs are a consensus assessment of research findings that give guidance on what should be *done*, rather than a statement of what should be *achieved*.

CPGs are derived by consensus and represent recommendations for care—based on an appraisal of the evidence of intervention outcomes (NHMRC 2000a, 2000b). CPGs thus represent an efficient and meaningful way of guiding best practice. As such, they have become a prominent feature of EBHC practice.

A huge number of CPGs relating to wound care is now available. Practitioners in wound management have to sort out which of these CPGs are useful and which should be disregarded. A good starting-point for locating useful CPGs is to access the websites of reputable research organisations—such as the Cochrane Collaboration, the National Institute of Clinical Evidence, the Agency for Health Care Policy and Research (AHCPR), and the (Australian) National Health and Medical Research Council (NHMRC). Professional wound-care organisations, teaching hospitals, and relevant university departments are also reliable sources of information.

'It is important to check the level of evidence on which a particular guideline is based and how that evidence was obtained.'

If local wound-care practice appears to be different from that advised in CPGs, it is important to check the level of evidence on which a particular guideline is based and how that evidence was obtained. Weak levels of evidence are somewhat suspect, and changes to established practice should not necessarily be made on the basis of such evidence—especially if current practice is well established and apparently satisfactory.

If there is strong support for a suggested practice in guidelines *and* if local practice is different from the guidelines, change should be considered—but in a controlled fashion. In these circumstances, a comparative trial could be conducted so that local practice can be benchmarked before discarding it. If the guideline evidence is strong and current local practice is suspect, there is a good case for change.

'If there is strong support for a suggested practice in guidelines and if local practice is different from the guidelines, change should be considered.'

In addition to comparing local practice with published guidelines, such guidelines can be compared with each other. If practice recommendations vary from CPG to CPG, this might indicate poor levels of support for a given element of practice. In addition, some CPGs are better sourced than others. If there is no mention of the evidence-search strategy that has been used, the validity of the guidelines might be questionable.

Policies and procedures

Although CPGs are the most obvious (and perhaps best constructed) manifestations of best-practice principles, there are several other sources of guidance for best practice in the clinical setting. Hospitals, aged-care facilities, community-care providers, and wound-management clinics often create policies, procedures, consensus documents, clinical pathways, care algorithms, and standardised care plans in relation to wound management.

'Nurses are responsible for their own practice, and they therefore have a responsibility to ensure that local practice is always in accordance with current best practice.'

These documents are usually based on research evidence and/or historically accepted practices. As such, they fit nicely into the 'best-practice paradigm'.

Nurses should constantly apprise themselves of wound-management research to ensure that these documents continue to represent best practice and do not become outdated. Practice is always evolving, and changes will therefore occur over time. Nurses are responsible for their own practice, and they therefore have a responsibility to ensure that local practice is always in accordance with current best practice.

Conclusion

Best practice is synonymous with EBHC. Wound-management practice changes in accordance with research outcomes, and best practice thus implies keeping abreast of research outcomes and being able to adapt practice accordingly.

Research-based evidence is the most valuable evidence. CPGs provide an accessible form of research-based evidence, and can be used in the establishment of practice or for making relevant practice changes. Because CPGs are also subject to change according to new research, practitioners need to obtain updated versions as they become available.

Other documents—such as policies, procedures, consensus documents, clinical pathways, care algorithms, and standardised care plans—are also valuable in assessing best practice in relation to wound management. These should also be continually scrutinised and updated in accordance with research findings.

'If experience is coupled with research, the likely outcome is best practice.'

However, wound management is an art, as well as a science. Although most of the evidence used to develop CPGs and similar documents is derived from research, experience and other forms of information are also valuable. On occasions, a nurse's ability to adapt to different shaped limbs, different climates, or countless other variables can be the difference between best practice and poor practice. When used in isolation, personal experience might not provide best practice, but if experience is coupled with research, the likely outcome is best practice.

The nexus between evidence and experience can often best be articulated in *practice principles*. Principles lend themselves to adaptation, and this is ideal in the field of wound management. No two people are the same, and practice must account for individual differences.

'Principles lend themselves to adaptation, and this is ideal in the field of wound management ... no two people are the same.'

In summary, the necessary elements for best practice are: (i) continuous appraisal of the evidence; (ii) development of relevant guidelines and principles; (iii) comparison of personal experience with research results; and (iv) critique of current practice and its value to people with wounds.

References

Chapter I On Being Wounded

Bale, S. & Jones, V. 1997, *Wound Care Nursing: A Patient-Centred Approach*, Baillière Tindall, London.

Baxter, H. 2002, 'How a discipline came of age: a history of wound care', *Journal of Wound Care*, vol. 11, no. 10, pp 383–92.

Carville, K. 2001, *Wound Care Manual*, Silver Chain Foundation, Osborne Park, Western Australia.

Cullum, N. & Roe, B. 1998, *Leg Ulcers: Nursing Management A Research-based Guide*, Baillière Tindall, London.

Douglas, V. 2001, 'Living with a chronic leg ulcer: an insight into patients' experiences and feelings', *Journal of Wound Care*, vol. 10, no. 9, pp 355–60.

Edwards, L.M., Moffatt, C.J. & Franks, P.J. 2002, 'An exploration of patients' understanding of leg ulceration', *Journal of Wound Care*, vol. 11, no. 1, pp 35–9.

Jones, J. 1998, 'Compression, ulcer recurrence and compliance', *Journal of Wound Care (supplement)*,October, pp 9–13.

Lindsay, E. 2001, 'The social dimension in leg ulcer management', *Primary Intention*, vol. 9, no. 1, pp 31–3.

RCNA *see* Royal College of Nursing, Australia.

Royal College of Nursing, Australia) , 2000, *Position Statement: Quality in Nursing Practice*, <www.rcna.org.au/content/qualitynurspract.htm>.

Selim, P., Lewis, C. & Templeton, S. 2001, 'Evidence based practice and client compliance', *Journal of Community Nursing*, vol. 15, no. 5, pp 10–14.

Wattis, L., Mayhew, A. & Hillier, V. 1997, 'Research-based wound care: a fresh view of resistance to change', *Primary Intention*, vol. 5, no. 2, pp 35–9.

Chapter 2 The Skin and Healing

Carville, K. 2001, *Wound Care Manual*, 4th edn, Silver Chain Foundation, Western Australia.

Harding, K. 2001, *The Wound Care Programme*, Centre for Medical Education, Cardiff.

Tortora, G.J. 1997, *Introduction to the Human Body: The Essentials of Anatomy and Physiology*, 4th edn, Biological Sciences Textbooks, USA.

Winter, G.D. 1962, 'Formation of a scab and the rate of epithelialisation of superficial wounds in the skin of the young domestic pig', *Nature*, vol. 193, pp 293–4.

Chapter 3 Assessment and Documentation

Adderley, U. & Nelson, A. 2000, 'Know how: clinical photography', *Nursing Times*, 96 (45).

Australian Wound Management Association (AWMA) 2001, *Clinical Practice Guidelines for the Prediction and Prevention of Pressure Ulcers*, Cambridge Publishing, West Leederville, Western Australia.

Australian Wound Management Association (AWMA) 2002, *Standards for Wound Management*, Australian Wound Management Association.

AWMA *see* Australian Wound Management Association.

Bachand, P.M. & McNichols, M.E. 1999, 'Creating a wound assessment record', *Advances in Wound Care*, 12 (8), 426–9.

Bale, S. & Jones, V. 1997, *Wound Care Nursing: A patient-centred approach*, Bailliere Tindall, London.

Banks, V. 1998, 'Wound assessment methods', *Journal of Wound Care*, 7 (4), 211–12.

Benbow, M. 2002, 'The skin. Skin and wound assessment', *Nursing Times*, 98 (25), 41–4.

Carville, K. 2001, *Wound Care Manual*, Silver Chain Nursing Association, Osborne Park, Western Australia.

Dunford, C. 1999, 'Hypergranulation tissue', *Journal of Wound Care*, 8 (10), 506–7.

Fergusson, J.A.E. & MacLellan, D.G. 1997, 'Wound management in older people', *The Australian Journal of Hospital Pharmacy*, 27 (6).

Goldman, R.J. & Salcido, R. 2002, 'More than one way to measure a wound: an overview of tools and techniques', *Advances in skin and wound care*, 15 (5), 236–43.

Langemo, D.K., Melland, H., Hanson, D., Olson, B., Hunter, S. & Henly, S.J. 1998, 'Two-dimensional wound measurement: comparison of 4 techniques', *Advances in Wound Care*, 11 (7), 337–43.

Maklebust, J. & Sieggreen, M.Y. 2001, *Pressure ulcers: Guidelines for prevention and management*, Springhouse Corporation, Pennsylvania, USA.

Massie, T.J. 1998, 'Implemenation of change: a wound assessment chart', *Professional Nurse*, 14 (2), 118–22.

Morison, M., Moffatt, C., Bridel-Nixon, J. & Bale, S. 1997, *A Colour Guide to the Nursing Management of Chronic Wounds*, Mosby, London.

Pudner, R. 2002, 'Measuring Wounds', *Journal of Community Nursing*, 16 (9), 36–42.

Samad, A., Hayes, S., French, L. & Dodds, S. 2002, 'Digital imaging versus conventional contact tracing for the objective measurement for venous leg ulcers', *Journal of Wound Care*, 11 (4), 137–40.

Santamaria, N., Austin, D. & Clayton, L. 2002, 'A multi-site clinical evaluation trial of the Alfred/Medseed wound imaging system prototype', *Primary Intention*, 10 (3), 120–5.

Swann, G. 2000, 'Photography in wound care', *Nursing Times Plus*, 96 (7), 9–12.

Staunton, P.J. & Chiarella, M. 2003, *Nursing and the Law*, Churchill Livingstone, Sydney.

Templeton, S. 2003, 'Wound Assessment and Documentation', *The Pursuit of Excellence*, Royal District Nursing Service SA Inc., Issue 22, October 2003, <www.rdns.net.au/research_publications/Newsletters>.

Tennant, J. 2000, 'Care of the diabetic foot–assessment, treatment and management', *Woundcare Network*, Issue 4.

Thomas, S. 1997, 'Assessment and management of exudate', *Journal of Wound Care*, 6 (7), 327–30.

Williams, E. 1997, 'Assessing the Future', *Nursing Times*, 93 (23), 77–8.

Chapter 4 Dressings

Achterberg, V., Welling, C. & Meyer-Ingold, W. 1996, 'Hydroactive dressings and serum proteins: an *in vitro* study', *Journal of Wound Care*, vol. 5, no. 2.

Alderman, C. (ed) 2004a, 'Selected wound dressings—part one', *RGH Pharmacy E-bulletin*, vol. 12, no. 12.

Alderman, C. (ed) 2004b, 'Selected wound dressings—part two', *RGH Pharmacy E-bulletin*, vol. 13, no. 1.

Australian Wound Management Association 2002, *Standards for Wound Management*, Cambridge Publishing, West Leederville, Western Australia.

AWMA *see* Australian Wound Management Association.

Bolton, L.L., Van Rijswijk, L. & Shaffer, F.A. 1996, 'Quality wound care equals cost-effective wound care', *Nursing Management*, vol. 27, no. 7.

Carmody, S. & Forster, S. (eds) 2003, *Aged Care Nursing: A Guide to Practice*, Ausmed Publications, Melbourne.

Carville, K. 2001, *The Wound Care Manual*, Silver Chain Nursing Association, Osborne Park, Western Australia.

Collins, F., Hampton, S. & White, R. 2002, *A–Z Dictionary of Wound Care*, Quay Books, Wiltshire, England.

ConvaTec, 1998, *Solutions from ConvaTec: Wound and Skin Management System. A guide to caring for your wound* (pamphlet).

ConvaTec, 1999, <www.convatec.com/wound2/healing/wscase1.htm>.

Falanga, V. 1997, 'Iodine-containing pharmaceuticals: a reappraisal', *Proceedings of the 6th European Conference on Advances in Wound Management*, Macmillan Magazines Ltd, London.

Jones, V. & Milton, T. 2000a, 'When and how to use adhesive film dressings', *Nursing Times Plus*, vol. 96, no. 14, pp 3–4.

Jones, V. & Milton, T. 2000b, 'When and how to use foam dressings', *Nursing Times Plus*, vol. 96, no. 36, pp 2–3.

Jones, V. & Milton, T. 2000c, 'When and how to use iodine dressings', *Nursing Times Plus*, vol. 96, no. 45, pp 2–3.

Lansdown, A.B.G. 2002, 'Silver I: its antibacterial properties and mechanism of action', *Journal of Wound Care*, vol. 11, no. 4, pp 125–9.

MacLellan, D.G. & Rice, J. 1995, 'Modern wound dressings in acute trauma', *Veterans' Health*, March.

Parnham, A. 2002, 'Moist wound healing: does the theory apply to chronic wounds?' *Journal of Wound Care*, vol. 11, no. 4, pp 143–6.

Pudner, R. 1997, 'Choosing an appropriate wound dressing', *Journal of Community Nursing*, vol. 11, no. 9, pp 34–9.

Sibbald, G., Williamson, D., Orsted, H.L., Campbell, K., Keast, D., Krasner, D. & Sibbald, D. 2000, 'Preparing the wound bed—debridement, bacterial balance and moisture balance', *OstomyWound Management*, vol. 46, no. 11, pp 14–35.

Templeton, S. 2001, 'Reviewing the use of honey on wounds', *The Pursuit of Excellence*, RDNS Research Unit, <www.rdns.net.au/research_publications/newsletter/01_woundmanagement_nov01.pdf>.

Thomas, S. 2003, 'Atraumatic dressings', *World Wide Wounds*, <www.worldwidewounds.com/2003/january/thomas/atraumatic-dressings.html>.

Winter, G.D. 1962, 'Formation of the scab and the rate of epithelialisation of superficial wounds in the skin of the young domestic pig', *Nature*, vol. 193, no. 4812, pp 293–4.

Wright, J.B., Lam, K. & Burrell, R.E. 1998, 'Wound management in an era of increasing bacterial antibiotic resistance: A role for topical silver treatment', *American Journal of Infection Control*, vol. 26, no. 6, pp 572–7.

World Union of Wound Healing Societies 2004, *Minimising pain at wound dressing-related procedures: A consensus document*, Medical Education Partnership Ltd, London.

WUWHS *see* World Union of Wound Healing Societies.

Chapter 5 Cleansing and Skin Care

Bergstrom,N., Allman, R.M., Alvarez, O., Bennett, M.A., Carlson, C.E. & Frantz, R.A. 1994, *Treatment of pressure ulcers. Clinical practice guideline, No. 15*, Public Health Service, Agency for Health Care Policy and Research, AHCPR Publication No. 95-052.

Blunt, J. 2001, 'Wound cleansing: ritualistic or research-based practice', *Nursing Standard*, 16(1), 33–6.

Burks, R. 1998, 'Povidone-Iodine Solution in Wound Treatment', *Physical Therapy*, 78, 212–18.

Cochrane Library 2002, *Water for Wound Cleansing*, Issue 1.

Cooper, R. 2004, 'A review of the evidence for the use of topical antimicrobial agents in wound care', *World Wide Wounds*, 1–14.

Crow, S. 1997, 'Infection control perspectives', in Krasner, D. & Kane, D. (eds), *Chronic Wound Care*, 2, 90–6.

Dealey, C. 1994, *The Care of Wounds*, Blackwell Scientific Publications, Oxford.

Faller, N.A. 1997, 'A survey exploring the ET nursing art of wound care: Factors associated with clean versus sterile technique', unpublished PhD thesis, University of Massachusetts.

Fernandez, R., Griffiths, R. & Ussia, C. 2002, *The Effectiveness of Solutions, Techniques and Pressure in Wound Cleansing: A systematic review*, The Joanna Briggs Institute for Evidence Based Nursing and Midwifery.

Karukonda, S., Corcoran,T., Erin, B., McBurney, E., Russo, G. & Millikan, L. 2000, 'The effects of drugs on wound healing: Part 2', *International Journal of Dermatology*, 39(5), 321–33.

Lawrence, J.C. 1998, 'The use of iodine as an antiseptic agent', *Journal of Wound Care*, 7(8), 421–5.

Leaper, D. 1996, 'Antiseptics in wound healing', *Nursing Times*, 92, 63–4.

Lineweaver, W. 1985, 'Topical antimicrobial toxicity', *Archives of Surgery*, 120, 267–70.

Morison, M. 1992, 'Wound cleansing: Which Solution?' in *A Colour Guide to the Nursing Management of Wounds*, Wolfe Publishing Ltd, London, p. 51.

Morison, M. 1998, *Nursing Management of Chronic Wounds*, Mosby.

Oliver, L. 1997, 'Wound Cleansing', *Nursing Standard*, 11 (20), 47–56.

Ovington, L.G. 2001, 'Battling Bacteria in Wound Care', *Home Healthcare Nurse*, 19 (10), 622–30.

Pirnay, J.P., De Vos, D., Cochez, C., Bilocq, F., Pirson, J. & Struelens, M. 2000, 'A molecular epidemiology of *pseudomonas aeruginosa* colonization in a burn unit: persistence of a multidrug-resistance clone and a silver sulfadiazine-resistant clone', *Journal of Clinical Microbiology*, 41(3), 1192–202.

Stotts, N.A., Barbour, S., Griggs, K., Bouvier, B., Buhlman, L. & Wipke-Tevis, D. 1997, 'Sterile versus clean technique in postoperative wound care of patients with open surgical wounds: a pilot study', *Journal of Wound Care*, 24, 10–18.

Thomlinson, D. 1987, 'To clean or not to clean?' *Nursing Times*, 83 (9), 71–5.

Williams, C. 1999, 'Wound irrigation techniques: new Steripod normal saline', *British Journal of Nursing*, 8(21), 1460–2.

Young, T. 1995, 'Common problems in wound care: wound cleansing', *British Journal of Nursing*, 4(5), 286–9.

Chapter 6 Wound Bed Preparation

Ayello, E. & Cuddigan, J.E., 2004, 'Debridement: controlling the necrotic/cellular burden', *Advances in Skin & Wound Care*, 17(2): 66–75.

Chin, C., Schultz, G., Stacey, M., Falanga, V., Sibbald, G., Dowsett, C., Harding, K., Romanelli, M., Teot, L. & Vanscheidt, W. 2003, 'Principles of wound bed preparation and their application to the treatment of chronic wounds', *Primary Intention*, 11(4): 171–82.

Edwards, R. & Harding, K. 2004, 'Bacteria and wound healing', *Current Opinion in Infectious Diseases*, 17: 91–6.

Enoch, S. & Harding, K. 2003, 'Wound bed preparation: The science behind the removal of barriers to healing', *Wounds*, 15(7): 213–29.

Fairbairn, K., Grier, J., Hunter, C. & Preece, J. 2002, 'A sharp debridement procedure devised by specialist nurses', *Journal of Wound Care*, 11(10): 371–5.

Flanagan, M. 2003, 'The philosophy of wound bed preparation in clinical practice', *Wound Bed Preparation*, Smith & Nephew Medical Ltd, 1–34.

Grayson, M.L., Gibbons, G.W., Balogh, K., Levin, E. & Karchmer, A.W. 1995, 'Probing to bone in infected pedal ulcers: A clinical sign of underlying osteomyelitis in diabetic patients', *Journal of the American Medical Association*, 273(9): 721–3.

Hess, C.T. & Kirsner, R.S. 2003, 'Orchestrating wound healing: Assessing and preparing the wound bed', *Advances in Skin & Wound Care*, 16(5): 246–57.

LarvE, 2003, 'Mechanisms of action', <www.larve.com/maggot_manual>, October.

Leaper, D. 2002, 'Sharp technique for wound debridement', <www.worldwidewounds.com>.

Ramundo, J. & Wells, J. 2000, 'Wound Debridement', in Bryant, R. (ed.), *Acute & Chronic Wounds: Nursing Management*, 2nd edn, Mosby Inc., St Louis.

Schultz, G.S., Sibbald, G.R., Falanga, V., Ayello, E., Dowsett, C., Harding, K., Romanelli, K., Stacey, M., Teot, L. & Vanscheidt, W. 2003, 'Wound Bed Preparation: a systematic approach to wound management', *Wound Repair and Regeneration*, 11(2): 1–28.

Sibbald, G.R., Orstead, H., Shultz, G.S., Coutts, P. & Keast, D. 2003, 'Preparing the Wound Bed 2003: Focus on Infection and Inflammation', *Ostomy/Wound Management*, 49(11): 24–51.

Chapter 7 Nutrition and Healing

Bartlett, S., Marian, M., Taren, D. & Muramoto, M. 1998, *Geriatric Nutrition Handbook*, Chapman and Hall Nutrition Handbooks 5, Thomson Publishing, New York.

Carmody, S. & Forster, S. 2003, *Aged Care Nursing: A Guide to Practice*, Ausmed Publications, Melbourne.

Chang, B. 1997, *The TwoCal HN Med Pass Program: A Medically Effective Cost-Avoidance Tool for Long-Term Care Facilities in a Managed Care*, Era Ross Products Division, Abbott Laboratories, 11: 1–4.

Escott-Stump, S. 1998, *Nutrition and Diagnosis-related Care*, 4th edn, Williams and Wilkins, Baltimore, pp 77–9.

Ferguson, M., Cook, A., Rimmasch, H., Bender, S. & Voss, A. 2000, 'Pressure ulcer management: The importance of nutrition', *Medsurg Nursing*, vol. 9, no. 4, pp 163–7.

Schmidt, T.R. 2002, *Wound care in long-term care: What's new in Nutrition?*, Extended Care Product News 81: 18–20.

Chapter 8 Trauma

Australian Wound Management Association 2002, *Standards for Wound Management*, AWMA, Perth.

AWMA, see Australian Wound Management Association.

Blank-Reid, C. 2004, 'Abdominal trauma', *Nursing*, 34(9), 36–41.

Cuzzell, J. 2002, 'Wound assessment and evaluation: Skin tear protocol', *Dermatology Nursing*, 14(6), 405.

Everett, S. & Powell, T. 1994, 'Skin tears—the underestimated wound', *Primary Intention*, 2(1), 28–30.

Gilchrest, B.A. 1982, 'Age-associated changes in the skin', *Journal of the American Geriatrics Society*, 139–43.

Kaminer, M.S. & Gilchrest, B.A. 1994, 'Aging of the skin', in W. Hazzard (ed.), *Principles of Geriatric Medicine and Gerontology*, pp 411–15, McGraw-Hill, New York.

Kurt, N., Fehmi Kucuk, H., Demirhan, R. & Altaca, G. 2003, 'Crush injury in two earthquake disasters within a 3-month period', *European Journal of Trauma*, 29(1), 42–5.

Laskowski-Jones, L. 2002, 'Responding to an out-of-hospital emergency', *Nursing*, 32(9), 36–43.

McGough-Csarny, J. & Kopac, C.A. 1998, 'Skin tears in institutionalized elderly: an epidemiological study', *Ostomy Wound Management*, 44(3A), 14S–25S, 38S–40S.

McGregor, I.A. 1990, *Fundamental Techniques of Plastic Surgery*, Churchill Livingstone, Edinburgh.

Meulenieire, F. 2003, 'The management of skin tears', *Nursing Times*, 99(5), S69–71.

O'Regan, A. 2002, 'Skin tears: A review of the literature', *World Council of Enterostomal Therapists Journal*, 22(2), 26–31.

Payne, R.L. & Martin, M. 1990, 'The epidemiology and management of skin tears in older adults', *Ostomy Wound Management*, 26, 26–37.

Payne, R.L. & Martin, M. 1993, 'Defining and classifying skin tears: Need for a common language. A critique and revision of the Payne–Martin classification system for skin tears', *Ostomy Wound Management*, 39(5), 16–20.

Pignone, M. & Levin, B. 2002, 'Information from your family doctor: Caring for cuts, scrapes, and wounds', *American Family Physician*, 66(2), 315–16.

Silva, A.J. 1999, 'Mechanism of injury in gunshot wounds: Myths and reality', *Critical Care Nursing Quarterly*, 22(1), 69–74.

Singer, A.J., Hollander, J.E. & Quinn, J.V. 1997, 'Evaluation and management of traumatic lacerations', *The New England Journal of Medicine*, 337(16), 1142–8.

Steffen, K.A. 2003, 'When your trauma patient is over', *Nursing*, 33(4), 53–6.

Templeton, S. 2003, *Promoting evidence-based nursing practice: Older people and skin tears*, Royal District Nursing Service Research Unit, Adelaide.

Waller, R. (ed.) 2004, *Wound Care and Repair*, 2nd edn, Churchill Livingstone, Sydney.

White, M.W., Karam, S. & Cowell, B. 1994, 'Skin tears in frail elders: A practical approach to prevention', *Geriatric Nursing*, 15, 95–9.

Chapter 9 Reconstructive Techniques

Argenta, L.C. & Morykwas, M.J. 1997, 'Vacuum-assisted closure: A new method for wound control and tratment: Clinical Experience', *Annals of Plastic Surgery*, 38(6), 563–76.

Banwell, P. E. 1999, 'Topical negative pressure therapy in wound care', *Journal of Wound Care*, 8(2), 79–84.

Banwell, P.E. & Teot, L. 2003, 'Topical negative pressure (TNP): The evolution of a novel wound therapy', *Journal of Wound Care*, 12(1).

Clamon, J. & Netscher, D.T. 1994, 'General principles of flap reconstruction: Goals for aesthetic and functional outcome', *Plastic Surgical Nursing*, 14(1), 9–13.

Deva, A.K., Buckland, G.H., Fisher, E., Liew, S.C.C., Merten, S., McGlynn, M., et al. 2000, 'Topical negative pressure in wound management', *Medical Journal of Australia*, 173, 128–31.

Dinman, S. & Giovannone, M.K. 1994, 'The care and feeding of microvascular flaps: How nurses can prevent flap loss', *Plastic Surgical Nursing*, 14(3), 154–64.

Francis, A. 1998, 'Nursing management of skin graft sites', *Nursing Standard*, 12(33), 41–4.

Grabb, W.C. & Smith, J.W. (eds) 1979, *Plastic Surgery*, 3rd edn, Little, Brown and Co., Boston.

Kane, D.P. 1997, 'Surgical Repair', in D. Krasner & D.P. Kane (eds.), *Chronic Wound Care: A clinical source book for health professionals*, 2nd edn, Health Management Publications, Wayne.

Maksud, D.P. 1992, 'Nursing management of patients following combined free flap mandible reconstruction', *Plastic Surgical Nursing*, 12(3), 95–105.

Maksud-Sagrillo, D. & Mooney, K.M. 1999, 'Advances in wound closure techniques', *Plastic Surgical Nursing*, 19(4), 208–9.

McGregor, I.A. 1989, *Fundamental Techniques of Plastic Surgery and their Surgical Applications*, 8th edn, Churchill Livingstone, Edinburgh.

Mendez-Eastman, S.K. 2001, 'Skin Grafting: Preoperative, intraoperative, and postoperative care', *Plastic Surgical Nursing*, 21(1), 49–51.

Morykwas, M.J., Argenta, L.C. & Winton-Salem, N.C. 1997, 'Nonsurgical modalities to enhance healing and care of soft tissue wounds', *Journal of Southern Orthopaedic Association*, 6(4), 279–88.

Sandau, K.E. 2002, 'Free TRAM flap breast reconstruction', *American Journal of Nursing*, 102(4), 36–42.

Schneider, A.M. Morykwas, M.J. & Argenta, L.C. 1998, 'A new and reliable method of securing skin grafts to the difficult recipient bed', *Journal of Plastic and Reconstructive Surgery*, 102(4), 1195–8.

Chapter 10 Leg Ulcers

Anderson, I. 1995, 'Doppler ultrasound recording of ankle brachial pressure index in the community', *Journal of Wound Care*, vol. 4, no.7, pp 325–7.

Carville, K. 2001, *Wound Care Manual*, Silver Chain Foundation, Osborne Park, Western Australia.

Cullum, N. & Roe, B. 1998, *Leg Ulcers: Nursing Management—A research-based guide*, Baillière Tindall, London.

Dowsett, C. 2001, 'Leg ulcer management: Leg ulcer skin care', *Journal of Wound Care*, vol. 10, no. 4 (supplement).

Harker, J. 2002, 'Promoting best practice in leg ulcer assessment', *Nursing Times*, vol. 98, no. 44, pp 60–1.

Hewitt, A., Flesker, R., Harcourt, D. & Sinha, S. 2003, 'The evolution of a hospital-based leg ulcer clinic', *Primary Intention*, vol. 11, no. 2, pp 75–85.

Hislop, 1997, 'Leg ulcer assessment by Doppler ultrasound', *Nursing Standard*, vol. 11, no. 43, pp 49–56.

Iannos, J. 1998, 'Ankle brachial pressure index and assessment of arterial occlusive disease', *Journal of Stomal Therapy*, vol. 18, no. 4, pp 10–12.

Mear, J. & Moffatt, C. 2002, 'Bandaging technique in the treatment of venous ulcer', *Nursing Times*, vol. 98, no. 44, pp. 44–6.

Morison, M., Moffatt, C., Bridel-Nixon, J. & Bale, S. 1997, *Nursing Management of Chronic Wounds*, Mosby, London.

Morris, D. & Kerstein, M.D. 2001, 'Lower extremity wounds. 1: Vascular disease assessment', *Journal of Wound Care*, vol. 10, no.10, pp 395–8.

Nelson, E.A., Ruckley, C.V., Dale, J. & Morison, M. 1996, 'The management of leg ulcers', *Journal of Wound Care*, vol. 5, no. 2, pp 73–6.

RCN *see* Royal College of Nursing Institute (UK).

Rice, K. 1998, 'Navigating a bottleneck', *Nursing 98*, February, pp 33–8.

Royal College of Nursing Institute (UK) 1998, *Clinical Practice Guidelines: The Management of Patients with Venous Leg Ulcers*, <www.rcn.org.uk/publications/pdf/guidelines/venous_leg_ulcers.pdf>.

Scottish Intercollegiate Guidelines Network 1998, *The Care of Patients with Chronic Leg Ulcer*, <www.show.scot.nhs.uk/sign/pdf/sign26.pdf>.

Scully, C. 1999, 'In on a limb', *Nursing Times*, 95(27): 59–65.

SIGN *see* Scottish Intercollegiate Guidelines Network.

Smith, D. 2002, 'The management of mixed arterial ulcers', *Woundcare Network*, issue 8, July.

Thomas, C. 1998, 'Caring for venous ulcers', *Nursing 98*, September, p. 18.

Vowden, K. 1998, 'Lipodermatosclerosis and atrophie blance', *Journal of Wound Care*, vol. 7, no. 9, pp 441–3.

Vowden, P. 1998, 'The investigations and assessment of venous disease', *Journal of Wound Care*, vol. 7, no. 3, pp 143–7.

Vowden, K. & Vowden, P. 1996a, 'Hand-held doppler assessment for peripheral arterial disease', *Journal of Wound Care*, vol. 5, no. 3, pp 125–8.

Vowden, K. & Vowden, P. 1996b, 'Peripheral arterial disease', *Journal of Wound Care*, vol. 5, no. 1, pp. 23–6.

Vowden, K. & Vowden, P. 2001, 'Doppler and the ABPI: how good is our understanding?', *Journal of Wound Care*, vol. 10, no. 6, pp 197–202.

Chapter 11 Bandaging and Compression Therapy

Carville, K. 2001, *Wound Care Manual*, Silver Chain Foundation, Osborne Park, Western Australia.

Cullum, N. & Roe, B. 1998, *Leg Ulcers: Nursing Management, A Research Based Guide*, Bailliére Tindall, London.

Cullum, N., Fletcher, A.W., Nelson, E. A. & Sheldon, T.A. 1998, 'Compression bandages and stockings in the treatment of venous leg ulcers', *The Cochrane Library*, Issue 4.

Fletcher, A., Cullum, N. & Sheldon, T.A. 1997, 'A systematic review of compression treatment for venous leg ulcers', *British Medical Journal*, vol. 315, September, pp 576–80.

Hampton, S. 1998, 'Bandage application', *Journal of Wound Care* (supplement), October.

Harker, J. 2002, 'Promoting best practice in leg ulcer assessment', *Nursing Times Plus*, vol. 98, no. 44, pp 60–1.

Hewitt, A., Flekser, R., Harcourt, D. & Sinha, S. 2003, 'The evolution of a hospital-based leg ulcer clinic', *Primary Intention*, vol. 11. no. 2, pp 75–85.

Hofman, D. 1998, 'Oedema and its treatment', *Journal of Wound Care* (supplement), July.

Jones, J. 1998, 'Compression, ulcer recurrence and compliance', *Journal of Wound Care* (supplement), October.

Mear, J. & Moffatt, C. 2002, 'Bandaging technique in the treatment of venous ulcers', *Nursing Times Plus*, vol. 98, no. 44, pp 44–6.

Morison, M. & Moffatt, C. 1994, *A Colour Guide to the Assessment and Management of Leg Ulcers*, Mosby, London.

Negus, D. 1991, *Leg Ulcers: A Practical Approach to Management*, Butterworth-Heinemann, Oxford.

Nelson, E. A. 1996, 'Compression bandaging in the treatment of venous leg ulcers', *Journal of Wound Care*, vol. 5, no. 9, pp 417–18.

Nelson, A. & Thomas, S. 1998, 'Selecting bandages', *Journal of Wound Care* (supplement), September.

NHS *see* NHS Centre for Reviews and Dissemination.

NHS Centre for Reviews and Dissemination, (University of York) 1997, 'Compression therapy for venous leg ulcers', *Effective Health Care*, vol. 3, no. 4, pp 1–12.

RCN Institute (Royal College of Nursing UK), 1998, *Clinical Practice Guidelines: The Management of Patients with Venous Leg Ulcers*, <www.rcn.org.uk/publications/pdf/guidelines/venous_leg_ulcers.pdf>.

Rice, J. 2002, 'Handy hints when treating venous leg ulcers and using compression therapy', *Primary Intention*, vol. 10, no. 3, pp 129–34.

Scottish Intercollegiate Guidelines Network 1998, *The Care of Patients with Chronic Leg Ulcer*, <www.show.scot.nhs.uk/sign/pdf/sign26.pdf>.

SIGN *see* Scottish Intercollegiate Guidelines Network.

Smith & Nephew 2002, *Profore: Four Layer Bandage System. Guidelines: Venous Leg Ulcer Treatment.*

Stacey, M. 2002, 'Compression therapy in the treatment of venous leg ulcers', *Nursing Times Plus*, vol. 98, no. 36, pp. 39–43.

Stacey, M., Falanga, V., Marston, W., Moffatt, Phillips, Sibbald, Vanscheidt, W. & Lindholm, C. 2002, 'The use of compression therapy for the treatment of venous leg ulcers: A recommended management pathway', *EWMA (European Wound Management Association) Journal*, vol. 2, no. 1, pp 3–7.

Stockport, J.C., Groarke, B.A., Ellison, D. A. & McCollum, C. 1997, 'Single-layer and multilayer bandaging in the treatment of venous leg ulcers', *Journal of Wound Care*, vol. 6, no. 10, pp 485–8.

Thomas, S. 1996, 'High compression bandages', *Journal of Wound Care*, vol. 5, no. 1. pp 40–3.

Thomas, S. & Nelson, A. 1998a, 'Graduated external compression in the treatment of venous disease', *Journal of Wound Care* (supplement), September.

Thomas, S. & Nelson, A. 1998b, 'Types of compression bandage', *Journal of Wound Care* (supplement), September.

Vowden, K. & Vowden, P. 1998, 'Anatomy, physiology and venous ulceration', *Journal of Wound Care* (supplement), July.

Chapter 12 Pressure Ulcers

Allman, R.M., Laprade, C.A., Noel, L.B., Walker, J.M., Moorer, C.A., Dear, M.R. & Smith, C.R. 1986, 'Pressure sores among hospitalised patients', *Annals of Internal Medicine*, 105(3): 337–342.

Alterescue, V. & Alterescue, K.B. 1992, 'Pressure ulcers: Assessment and treatment', *Orthopaedic Nursing*, 11(2): 37–49.

Anderson, K.E. & Kvorning, S.A. 1982, 'Medical aspects of the decubitus ulcer', *International Journal of Dermatology*, 21: 265–70.

Andrychuk, M.A. 1998, 'Pressure ulcers: Causes, risk factors, assessment, and intervention', *Orthopaedic Nursing*, 17(4): 65–81.

Australian Wound Management Association 2001, *Clinical Practice Guidelines for the Prediction and Prevention of Pressure Ulcers*, Cambridge Publishing, West Leederville WA.

AWMA *see* Australian Wound Management Association.

Bates-Jensen, B.M. 1998, 'Pressure Ulcers: pathophysiology and prevention', in Sussman, C. & Bates-Jensen, B.M. (eds), *Wound Care: A Collaborative Practice Manual for Physical Therapists and Nurses*, Aspen Publishers, Maryland.

Bergstrom, N., Bennett, M.A., Carlson, C.E., et al. 1994, *Treatment of Pressure Ulcers*, Clinical Practice Guideline No. 15, Rockville, MD: US Department of Health and Human Services, Public Health Service, Agency for Health Care Policy and Research. AHCPR No 95-0652.

Bergstrom, N., Braden, B.J., Laguzza, A. & Holman, V. 1987, 'The Braden Scale for predicting pressure sore risk', *Nursing Research*, 36(4): 205–10.

Bethell, E. 1994, 'The development of a strategy for the prevention and management of pressure sores', *Journal of Wound Care*, 3(7): 342–3.

Black, J.M. & Black, S.B. 1987, 'Surgical Management of Pressure Ulcers'. *Nursing Clinics North America*, 22(2): 429–38.

Bliss, M.R. 1998, 'Pressure injuries: causes and prevention', *Hospital Medicine*, 59(11): 841–4.

Braden, B. & Bergstrom, N. 1987, 'A conceptual schema for the study of the etiology of pressure sores', *Rehabilitation Nursing*, 12(1): 8–16.

Bridel, J. 1993, 'Assessing the risk of pressure sores', *Nursing Standard*, 7(5): 32–5.

Bryant, R.A., Shannon, M.L., Pieper, B., Braden, B.J. & Morris, D.J. 1992, 'Pressure Ulcers', in Bryant, R.A. *Acute and Chronic Wounds–Nursing Management*, Mosby, St Louis.

Burd, C., Langemo, D.K., Olson, B., Hanson, D., Hunter, S. & Sauvage. T. 1992, 'Skin problems: Epidemiology of pressure ulcers in a skilled care facility', *Journal of Gerontological Nursing*, 18(9): 29–39.

Clark, M. 2002, 'Pressure ulcers and quality of life', *Nursing Standard*, 13(16): 74–80.

Clark M. & Callum N. 1992, 'Matching patient need for pressure sore prevention with supply of pressure redistributing mattresses', *Journal of Advanced Nursing*, 17: 310–16.

Cograve, M., West, H. & Leonard, B. 2002, 'Topical negative pressure for pressure ulcer management', *British Journal of Nursing*, 11(6): S29–S36.

Colburn, L. 1990, 'Early intervention for the prevention of pressure ulcers', in Krasner, D. (ed.), *Chronic wound care: A clinical source book for health professionals*, King of Prussia Health Management Publications Inc., Philadelphia.

Cooper, D.M. 1992, 'Wound assessment and evaluation', in Bryant, R.A. (ed.), *Acute and Chronic Wound Care: Nursing Management.* Mosby, St Louis.

Crest 1998, 'Crest Guidelines for the Prevention and Management of Pressure Sores: Recommendations for Practice', Belfast, Ireland 1998, <www.crestni.org.uk/publications/pressure_sores.pdf>.

Culley, F. 1998, 'Nursing aspects of pressure sore prevention and therapy', *British Journal of Nursing*, 7(15): 879–86.

Dinsdale, S.M. 1974, 'Decubitus ulcers: Role of pressure and friction in causation', *Archives of Physical Medical Rehabilitation*, 55:147-152.

Eaglestein, W.H. & Falanga, V. 1997, 'Chronic wounds', *Surgical Clinics North America*, 77(3): 689–700.

Edberg, E., Cerny, K. & Stauffer, E. 1973, 'Prevention and Treatment of Pressure Sores', *Physical Therapy*, 53(3): 246–52.

Exton-Smith, A.M. & Sherwin, R.W. 1961, 'The Prevention of Pressure Sores— Significance of spontaneous bodily movements', *The Lancet*, 18: 1124–6.

Feedar, J.A. 1995, 'Prevention and management of pressure ulcers', in McCullough, J.M., Kloth L.C. & Feeder, J.A. (eds), *Wound Healing: alternatives in management*, F.A. Davis, Philadelphia.

Flanagan, M. 1993, 'Pressure sore risk assessment scales', *Journal of Wound Care*, 2(3):162-167.

Frantz, R. 2004, 'Evidence-Based Protocol: Prevention of Pressure Ulcers', *Journal of Gerontological Nursing*, 30(2): 4–11.

Hamilton, F. 1992, 'An analysis of the literature pertaining to pressure sore risk assessment scales', *Journal of Clinical Nursing*, 1(4): 185–93.

Harding, K. & Boyce, D.E. 1998, 'Wounds: the extent of the burden', in Leaper, D.J. & Harding, K., *Wounds: Biology and Management*, Oxford University Press, Oxford.

Henderson, C.T., Ayello, E.A., Sussman, C., Leiby, D.M., Bennett, M.A., Dungong, E.F., Sprigle, S. & Woodruff, L. 1997, 'Draft Definition of Stage 1 pressure ulcers: inclusion of persons with darkly pigmented skin, NPUAP Task Force on Stage 1 and Darkly Pigmented Skin', *Advances in Wound Care*, 10(5): 16–19.

Hitch, S. 1995, 'NHS Executive Nursing Directorate: Strategy for major clinical guidelines—Prevention and Management of Pressure Sores, A Literature Review', *J. Tissue Viability*, 5(1): 3–24.

Hirshberg, J., Rees, R.S., Marchant, B. & Dean, S. 2000, 'Osteomyelitis Related to Pressure Ulcers: The Cost of Neglect', *Advances in Skin & Wound Care*, 13(1): 25–9.

James, S. 1997, 'Pressure sores and mental health status', *Journal of Wound Care*, 6(10): 496–99.

Jolley, D., Wright, R., McGowan, S., Hickey, M.B., Campbell, D.A., Sinclair, R. & Montgomery, K.C. 2004, 'Preventing pressure ulcers with the Australian Medical Sheepskin: an open-label randomized controlled trial', *Medical Journal of Australia*, 180: 324–7.

Kane, D.P. 1997, 'Surgical repair', in Krasner, D. & Kane, D. (eds), 2nd edn, *Chronic Wound Care: A Clinical Source Book for Healthcare Professionals*, Health Management Publications, Wayne, PA.

Kenney, L. & Rithalia, S. 1999, 'Technical aspects of support surfaces', in 'Mattresses and Beds', *Journal of Wound Care Supplement*, Emap Healthcare, Luton.

Koziak, M. 1961, 'Etiology of decubitus ulcers', *Archives of Physical and Medical Rehabilitation*, 42: 19–29.

Krasner, D. 1997, 'Chronic wound pain', in Krasner, D. & Kane, D (eds), 2nd edn, *Chronic Wound Care: A Clinical Source Book for Healthcare Professionals*, Health Management Publications, Wayne, PA.

Krouskop, M. 1983, 'A synthesis of the factors which contribute to pressure sore formation', *Medical Hypothesis*, 11: 255–67.

Lancet 1990, 'Preventing pressure sores', editorial, 2: 1311–12.

Longe, R.L. 1986, 'Current concepts in clinical therapeutics: Pressure sores', *Clinical Pharmacy*, 5: 669–81.

Makelebust, J. & Sieggreen, M. 1996, 'Etiology and pathophysiology of pressure ulcers', in *Pressure Ulcers—guidelines for prevention and nursing management*, Makelbust, J. & Sieggreen M. (eds), 2nd edn, Springhouse, Pennsylvania.

Michel, C.C. & Gillott, H. 1990, 'Microvascular mechanisms in stasis and ischaemia', in Bader, D.L. (ed.), *Pressure sores clinical practice and scientific approach*, Macmillan Press Ltd, London.

McGillick, J.M. 1990, 'Moving toward a patient care network: Social work and the pressure ulcer patient', in Krasner, D. (ed.), *Chronic Wound Care: A Clinical Source Book for Healthcare Professionals*, King of Prussia Health Management Publications Inc., Philadelphia.

National Institute for Clinical Excellence & National Collaboration Centre for Nursing and Supportive Care 2003, 'Clinical practice guideline for pressure-relieving devices: the use of pressure-relieving devices (beds, mattresses and overlays) for the prevention of pressure ulcers in primary and secondary care', <www.nice.org.uk/pdf/PRD_Fullguideline.pdf>.

National Pressure Ulcer Advisory Panel 1989, 'Pressure ulcers: incidence, economics, risk assessment. Consensus development conference statement', *Decubitus*, 2(2): 24–8.

National Pressure Ulcer Advisory Panel 1992, Panel for the Prediction and Prevention of Pressure Ulcers in Adults, *Pressure Ulcers in Adults: Prediction and Prevention. Clinical Practice Guideline, Number 3*, AHCPR Publication No. 92-0047, Rockville, MD: Agency for Health Care Policy and Research, Public Health Service, US Department of Health and Human Services.

NICE, *see* National Institute for Clinical Excellence & National Collaboration Centre for Nursing and Supportive Care.

NPUAP, *see* National Pressure Ulcer Advisory Panel.

Oot-Giromini, B.A. 1993, 'Pressure ulcer prevalence, incidence and associated risk factors in the community', *Decubitus*, 6(5): 24–32.

Porter, A. & Cooter, R. 1999, 'Surgical Management of Pressure Ulcers', *Primary Intention* 7(4): 151–5.

Reddy, N.P., Cochran, G.V. & Krouskop, T.A. 1980, 'Interstitial fluid as a factor in decubitus ulcer formation', *J. Biomechanics*, 14(12): 879–81.

Rund, C. 1997, 'Postoperative care of skin grafts, donor sites and myocutaneous flaps', in Krasner, D. & Kane, D. (eds), 2nd edn, *Chronic Wound Care: A Clinical Source Book for Healthcare Professionals*, Health Management Publications, Wayne, PA.

Rycroft-Malone, J. 2001, 'Pressure Ulcer Risk Assessment and Prevention Recommendations', Royal College of Nursing, London.

Scales, J.T. 1990, 'Pathogenesis of Pressure Sores', in Bader, D.L. (ed), *Pressure sores clinical practice and scientific approach*, MacMillan Press Ltd, London.

Shea, D.J. 1975, 'Pressure Sores', *Clinical Orthopaedics & Related Research*, 112: 89–101.

Shipperley, T. 1998, 'Guidelines for pressure sore prevention and management', *Journal of Wound Care*, 7(6): 309–11.

Smith, P.W., Black, J.M. & Black, S.B. 1999, 'Infected Pressure Ulcers in the Long-Term-Care Facility', *Infection Control and Hospital Epidemiology*, 20(5): 358–61.

Stotts, N.A. 1987, 'Age specific characteristics of patients who develop pressure ulcers in tertiary care settings', *Nursing Clinics of North America*, 22(2): 391–8.

Szor, J.K & Bourguignon, C. 1999, 'Description of pressure ulcer pain at rest and at dressing change', *Journal Wound Continence Ostomy Nurses*, 26(3): 115–20.

Thomas, D.R. 2001, 'Issues and Dilemmas in the Prevention and Treatment of Pressure Ulcers: A Review', *The Journals of Gerontology: Medical Sciences*, 56A(6): 328–40.

Torrance, C. 1983, *Pressure Sores: Aetiology, Treatment and Prevention*, Coom Helm, Beckenham.

Waterlow, J.A. 1988, 'The Waterlow Card for the prevention and management of pressure sores: Towards a pocket policy', *CARE-Science & Practice*, 6(1): 8–12.

Wellard, S. 2001, 'Mapping the management of pressure sores in SCI: An Australian case study', *SCI Nursing*, Publication of the American Association of Spinal Cord Injury Nurses, 18(1): 11–18.

Williams, C. 1993, 'Using water-filled gloves for pressure relief in heels', *Journal of Wound Care*, 2(6): 345–7.

Wysocki, A.B. & Bryant, R.A. 1992, 'Skin', in Bryant, R.A., *Acute and Chronic Wounds—Nursing Management*, Mosby, St Louis.

Young, J.B. & Dobranski, S. 1992, 'Pressure Sores. Epidemiology and Current Management Concepts', *Drugs & Ageing*, 2(1): 42–57.

Young, J. 1992, 'The use of specialised beds and mattresses', *Journal of Tissue Viability*, 2(3):79–81.

Young, Z.F., Evans, A. & Davis, J. 2003, 'Nosocomial Pressure Ulcer Prevention: A Successful Project', *Journal of Nursing Administration*, 33(7/8): 380–3.

Chapter 13 Burns

ANZBA *see* Australian and New Zealand Burn Association Ltd.

Australian and New Zealand Burn Association Ltd 2004, *Emergency Management of Severe Burns—Course Manual*, 7th edn.

Byers, J. & Flynn, M. 1996, 'Acute Burn Injury: A Trauma Case Report', *Critical Care Nurse*, vol 16, no. 4, pp 55–66.

Carrougher, G. 1998, 'Burn Wound Assessment and Topical Treatment', in Carrougher, G. (ed.), *Burn Care and Therapy*, Mosby, Missouri, pp 133–65.

Flannagan, M. & Graham, J. 2001, 'Should burn blisters be left intact or debrided?', *Journal of Wound Care*, vol. 10, no. 2, pp 41–5.

Jackson, D. 1953, 'The diagnosis of the depth of burning', *The British Journal of Surgery*, vol. 40, pp 588–96.

Lund, C.C. & Browder, N.C. 1944, 'The estimation of areas of burns', *Surgery, Gynaecology & Obstetrics*, vol. 79, pp 352–48.

Pankhurst, S. & Pochkhanawala, T. 2002, 'Wound Care', in Bosworth Bousfield, C. (ed.), *Burn Trauma Management & Nursing Care*, 2nd edn, Whurr Publishers, London, pp 81–108.

Williams, W. 2002, 'Pathophysiology of the burn wound', in Herndon, D. (ed) *Total Burn Care*, 2nd edn, Saunders, London, pp 514–21.

Chapter 14 Diabetes

Bowker, J.H. & Pfeifer, M.A. 2001, *Levin and O'Neals: The Diabetic Foot*, 6th edn, Mosby Year Book, St Louis.

McGill, M., Molyneaux, L. & Yue 1998, 'Use of the Semmes Weinstein 5.07/10gm monofilament: the long and short of it', *Diabetic Medicine*, 15: 615–17.

McGill, M., Molyneaux, L. & Yue, D. 2004, 'Which diabetic patients should receive podiatry care? An objective analysis', *Medical Journal of Australia* (forthcoming).

Thomson, F.J., Veves, A., Ashe, H. & Boulton, A.J.M. 1991, 'A team approach to diabetic footcare: the Manchester experience', *Foot*,1: 75–82.

Young, M.J., Cavanagh, P.R., Thomas, G., Johnson, M.N., Murray, H. & Boulton, A.J.M. 1992, 'Effect of callus removal on dynamic foot pressures in diabetic patients', *Diabetic Medicine*, 9: 75–7.

Chapter 15 Malignant Wounds

Back, I.N. & Finlay, I. 1995, 'Analgesic effect of topical opioids on painful skin ulcers' (letter), *Journal of Pain and Symptom Management*, 10(7): 493.

Collier, M. 1997, 'The assessment of patients with malignant fungating wounds—a holistic approach: part 2', *Nursing Times*, 93(46), Suppl. 1–4.

Collier, M. 2000, 'Management of patients with fungating wounds', *Nursing Standard*, 15 (11): 46–52.

Downing, J. 1999, *Pain in the Patient with Cancer, Nursing Times Clinical Monographs No 5*, NT Books, London.

Dunford, C. 2000, 'The use of honey in wound management', *Nursing Standard*, 15(11): 63–8.

Emflorgo, C. 1998, 'Controlling bleeding in fungating wounds' (letter), *Journal of Wound Care*, 7(5): 235.

Esther, R.J., Lamps, L. & Schwartz, H.S. 1999, 'Marjolin ulcers: secondary carcinomas in chromic wounds', *Journal of the Southern Orthopaedic Association*, 8(3): 181–7.

Flock, P., Gibbs, L. & Sykes, N. 2000, 'Diamorphine-metronidazole gel effective for treatment of painful infected leg ulcers' (letter), *Journal of Pain and Symptom Management*, 20(6): 396–7.

Gallagher, J. 1995, 'Management of cutaneous symptoms', *Seminars in Oncology Nursing*, 11(4): 239–47.

Grocott, P. 1995, 'Assessment of fungating malignant wounds', *Journal of Wound Care*, 4(7): 333–6.

Grocott, P. 1998, 'Controlling bleeding in fragile fungating tumours' (letter), *Journal of Wound Care*, 7(7): 342.

Grocott, P. 1999, 'The management of fungating wounds', *Journal of Wound Care*, 8(5): 232–4.

Grocott, P. 2000, 'Palliative management of fungating malignant wounds', *Journal of Community Nursing*, 14(3), 31-8.

Grocott, P. 2001, *Educational Booklet 8(2) The Palliative Management of Fungating Malignant Wounds*, Wound Care Society, Huntingdon, UK.

Haisfield-Wolfe, M.E. & Rund, C. 1997, 'Malignant cutaneous wounds: a management protocol', *Ostomy/Wound Management*, 43(1): 56–66.

Krajnik, M. & Zylicz, Z. 1997, 'Topical morphine for cutaneous cancer pain' (letter), *Palliative Medicine*, 11(4): 326.

Malheiro, E., Pinto, A., Choupina, M., Barroso, L., Reis, J. & Amarabte, J. 2001, 'Marjolin's ulcer of the scalp: case report and literature review', *Annals of Burns and Fire Disasters*, 14(1): <www.medbc.com/annals/review/vol_14/num_1/text/vol14n1p39.htm>.

Manning, M.P. 1998, 'Metastasis to skin', *Seminars in Oncology Nursing*, 14(3): 240–3.

Miller, C. 1998, 'Management of skin problems: nursing aspects', in Doyle, D., Hanks, G.W.C. & MacDonald, N. (eds), *Oxford Textbook of Palliative Medicine*, 2nd edn, pp. 642–56, Oxford University Press, Oxford.

Molan, P.C. 1999, 'The role of honey in the management of wounds', *Journal of Wound Care*, 8(8): 415–18.

Mortimer, P.S. 1998, 'Management of skin problems: medical aspects', in Doyle, D., Hanks, G.W.C. & MacDonald, N. (eds), *Oxford Textbook of Palliative Medicine*, 2nd edn, pp. 617–27, Oxford University Press, Oxford.

Naylor, W., Laverty, D. & Mallett, J. 2001, *The Royal Marsden Hospital Handbook of Wound Management in Cancer Care*, Blackwell Science Ltd, Oxford.

Naylor, W. 2002, 'Part 2: Symptom self-assessment in the management of fungating wounds', *World Wide Wounds*, <www.worldwidewounds.com/2002/july/Naylor-Part2/Wound-Assessment-Tool.html>

Newman, V., Allwood, M. & Oakes, R.A. 1989, 'The use of metronidazole gel to control the smell of malodorous lesions', *Palliative Medicine*, 34: 303–5.

Offer, G., Perks, G. & Wilcock, A. 2000, 'Palliative plastic surgery', *European Journal of Palliative Care*, 7(3): 85–7.

Pudner, R. 1998, 'The management of patients with a fungating or malignant wound', *Journal of Community Nursing*, 12(9): 30-4.

Stein, C. 1995, 'The control of pain in peripheral tissue by opioids', *The New England Journal of Medicine*, 332(25): 1685–90.

Thomas, S. 1992, *Current Practices in the Management of Fungating Lesions and Radiation Damaged Skin*, The Surgical Materials Testing Laboratory, Bridgend, Mid Glamorgan.

Thomas, S., Fischer, B., Fram, P.J. & Waring, M.J. 1998, 'Odour-absorbing dressings', *Journal of Wound Care*, 7(5): 246–50.

Thomas, S., Vowden, K. & Newton, H. 1998, 'Controlling bleeding in fragile fungating wounds', *Journal of Wound Care*, 7(3): 154.

Twillman, R.K., Long, T.D., Cathers, T.A. & Mueller, D.W. 1999, 'Treatment of painful skin ulcers with topical opioids', *Journal of Pain and Symptom Management*, 17(4): 288–92.

Van Toller, S. 1994, 'Invisible wounds: the effects of skin ulcer malodours', *Journal of Wound Care*, 3(2): 103–5.

WHO, *see* World Health Organization.

Wilkes, L., White, K., Smeal, T. & Beale, B. 2001, 'Malignant wound management: what dressings do nurses use?', *Journal of Wound Care*, 10(3): 65-70.

Williams, C. 1999, 'Clinisorb activated charcoal dressing for odour control', *British Journal of Nursing*, 8(15): 1016–19.

World Health Organization 1996, *Cancer Pain Relief*, 2nd edn, World Health Organization, Geneva.

Chapter 16 Draining Wounds, Fistulae, and Peristomal Wounds

Argenta L. & Morykwas, M. 1997, 'Vacuum-assisted closure: A new method for wound control and treatment—clinical experience' (reprint), *Annals of Plastic Surgery*, 38(6): 553–62.

Boyle, K., Fahl, R. & O'Brien, S. 1993, 'Don't double up', *Journal of Stomal Therapy*, 13(3): 8–11.

Brozenec, S. 1985, 'Caring for the postoperative patient with an abdominal drain', *Nursing*, 85, 15(4): 55–7.

Bryant, R. 1992, 'Management of drain sites and fistulas', in Bryant, R., *Acute and Chronic Wounds Nursing Management*, Mosby Year Book, St Louis.

Carville, K. 2001, *Wound Care Manual* , 4th edn, Silver Chain Foundation, Osborne Park, Western Australia.

Doughty, D. & Broadwell Jackson, D. 1993, *Gastrointestinal Disorders*, Mosby, St Louis.

Gray, M. & Jacobson, T. 2002, 'Are somatostatin analogues (octreotide and lanreotide) effective in promoting healing of enterocutaneous fistulas?', *Journal of Wound, Ostomy and Continence Nursing*, 29(5): 228–33.

Hardcastle, R. 1998, 'Vacuum-assisted closure therapy: The application of negative pressure in wound healing', *Primary Intention*, 6(1): 5–10.

Mattson Porth, C. 1986, *Pathophysiology Concepts of Altered Health States*, JB Lipincott, Philadelphia.

Ovington, L. 2002, 'Dealing with Drainage: The what, why and how of wound exudate', *Home Healthcare Nurse*, 20(6): 368–74.

Parnham, A. 2002. 'Moist wound healing: Does the theory apply to chronic wounds?', *Journal of Wound Care*, 11(4): 143–6.

Ratliff, C. & Donovan, A. 2001. 'Frequency of peristomal complications', *Ostomy Wound Management*, 47(8): 26–9.

Winter, G. 1962, 'Formation of the scab and the rate of epithelialisation of superficial wounds in the skin of the domestic pig', *Nature*, 193: 293–4.

Wysocki, A. 1996, 'Wound fluids and the pathogenesis of chronic wounds', *Journal of Wound, Ostomy and Continence Nursing*, 23(6): 283–90.

Chapter 17 Lymphoedema

Baumeister, R., Siuda, S., Bohmert, H. & Moser E. 1986, 'A microsurgical method for reconstruction of interrupted lymphatic pathway; ontologous lymph-vessel transplantation for treatment of lymphoedemas', *Scandinavian Journal of Plastic and Reconstructive Surgery and Hand Surgery*, vol. 20, pp 141–6.

Board, J. & Harlow, W. 2002, 'Lymphoedema', *British Journal of Nursing*, vol. 11, no. 7, pp 438–49.

Bellhouse, S. 2003, 'Simple Lymphatic Drainage', in Twycross, R., Jenns, K. & Todd, J. (eds), *Lymphoedema*, pp 217–35, Ausmed Publications, Melbourne.

BLS *see* British Lymphology Society.

British Lymphology Society 2001, *Clinical Definitions*, BLS, Sevenoaks, Kent.

Brorson, H., Svensson, H., Norrgren, K. & Throsson, O. 1998, 'Liposuction reduces arm lymphoedema without significantly altering the already impaired lymph transport', *Lymphology*, vol. 31, pp 156–72.

Carati, C.J., Anderson, S.N., Gannon, B.J. & Piller, N.B. 2003, 'Treatment of post-mastectomy lymphoedema with low-level laser therapy: double-blind, placebo-controlled trial', *Cancer*, vol. 98, pp 1114–22.

Piller, N. & Eaton, M. 2004, 'Lymphoedema optimizing outcomes', *Medicine Today*, vol. 5, November 4, pp 48–60.

Tortora, G.J. & Grabowski, S.R. (eds) 1996, 'The Lymphatic System, nonspecific resistance to disease and immunity', *Principles of Anatomy and Physiology*, 8th edn, Harper Collins, New York.

Weissleder, H. & Schuchhardt, C. 1997, *Lymphoedema Diagnosis and Therapy*, Kagerer Kommunication, Bonn, Germany.

Chapter 18 Dermatological Conditions

Budisavljevic, M.N., Cheek, D. & Ploth, D.W. 1996, 'Calciphylaxis in chronic renal failure', *Journal of the American Society of Nephrology*, 7(7): 978–82.

Callen, J.P. 1998, 'Pyoderma gangrenosum', *Lancet*, 351: 581–5.

Charles, J.J. & Falk, R.J. 1997, 'Medical progress: small-vessel vasculitis', *New England Journal of Medicine*, 337(21): 1512–23.

Chow, R.K.P. & Ho, V.C. 1996, 'Treatment of pyoderma gangrenosum', *Journal of American Academy of Dermatology*, 34: 1047–60.

DiNubile, M.J. & Lipsky, B.A. 2004, 'Complicated infections of skin and skin structures: when the infection is more than skin deep', *Journal of Antimicrobial Chemotherapy*, 53, Suppl. S2: ii 37–ii 50.

Ledbetter, L.S. Khoshnevis, M.R. & Hsu, S. 2000, 'Calciphylaxis', *Cutis*, 66(1): 49–53.

Lee, M. & Marks, R. 1998, 'The role of corticosteroids in dermatology', *Australian Prescriber*, (21): 9–11.

Machet, L., Couhe, C., Perrinaud, A., Hoaruau, C., Lorette, G., & Vaillant, L. 2004, 'A high prevalence of sensitisation persists in leg ulcer patient: a retrospective series of 106 patients tested between 2001 and 2002 and a meta-analysis of 1975–2003 data', *British Journal of Dermatology*, 150(5): 929–35.

Margolis, D.J. 1995, 'Management of unusual causes of ulcers of lower extremities', *Journal of Wound Ostomy and Continence Nursing*, 22: 89–94.

Mekkes, J.R., Loots, M.A.M., Vander Wall, A.C. & Bos, J.D. 2003, 'Causes, investigation and treatment of leg ulceration', *British Journal of Dermatology*, 148: 388–401.

Patel, G.H., Llewellyn, M., & Harding, K.G. 2001, 'Managing gravitational eczema and allergic contact dermatitis', *British Journal of Community Nursing*, 6(8): 394–406.

Shutler, S.D., Baragwanath, P., & Harding, K.G. 1995, 'Martorell's ulcer', *Postgraduate Medical Journal*, 71(842): 717–19.

Thompson, S.C., Jolley, D. & Marks, R. 1993, 'Reduction of solar keratosis by regular sunscreen use', *New England Journal of Medicine*, 329: 1147–51.

Von den Dreisch, P. 1997, 'Pyoderma gangrenosum: a report of 44 cases with follow-up', *British Journal of Dermatology*, 137: 1000–05.

Weening, R.H., Davis, M.D.H. & Dahl, P.R. 2002, 'Skin ulcers misdiagnosed as pyoderma gangrenosum', *New England Journal of Medicine*, 347: 1412–17.

Yang, D., Morrison, B.D., Vandogen, Y.K., Singh, A., & Stacey, M.C. 1996, 'Malignancy in chronic leg ulcers', *Medical Journal of Australia*, 164(12): 718–20:

Chapter 19 Best Practice

Bibbings, J. 1984, 'Honey, lizard dung and pigeon's blood', *Nursing Times*, November, 28: 36–8.

Carville, K. 1993, 'History of Wound Healing', *Primary Intention*, 1(1): 6–13.

Droogan, J. & Song, F. 1996, 'The process and importance of systematic reviews', *Nurse Researcher*, 4(1): 15–26.

Forbes, A. & Griffiths, P. 2002, 'Methodological strategies for the identification and synthesis of "evidence" to support decision-making in relation to complex healthcare systems and practices', *Nursing Inquiry*, 9(3): 141–55.

Greener, J. & Grimshaw, J. 1996, 'Using meta-analysis to summarise evidence within systematic reviews', *Nurse Researcher*, 4(1): 27–37.

Guyatt, G., Cook, D, & Haynes, B. 2004, 'Evidnce-based medicine has come a long way', *British Medical Journal*, 329 (7473): 990–1.

Johnson, A. 1988, 'Wound Management: Are you getting it right?', *The Professional Nurse*, May, 306–9.

Kitson, A. 2002, 'Recognising relationships: reflections on evidence-based practice', *Nursing Inquiry*, 9(3): 179–86.

Miller, B. & Keane, C. 1992, *Encyclopedia and Dictionary of Medicine, Nursing and Allied Health*, WB Saunders Company, Sydney.

National Health & Medical Research Council 1999, *A Guide To The Development, Implementation and Evaluation of Clinical Practice Guidelines*, NHMRC, Canberra.

National Health & Medical Research Council 2000a, *How to review the evidence: systematic identification and review of the scientific literature*, NHMRC, Canberra.

National Health & Medical Research Council 2000b, *How to use the evidence: assessment and application of scientific evidence*, NHMRC, Canberra.

NHMRC, *see* National Health & Medical Research Council.

Parker, J. 2002, 'Evidence-Based Nursing: A Defence', *Nursing Inquiry*, 9(3): 139–40.

Reed, J. & Procter, S. 1995, *Practitioner Research in Health Care*, Chapman and Hall, London.

Reilly, B. 2004, 'The essence of EBM', *British Medical Journal*, 329(7473): 991–2.

Sackett, D., Rosenberg, W., Muir-Gray, J.A., Haynes, R.B, Richardson, W.S. 1996, 'Evidence based medicine: what it is and what it isn't', *British Medical Journal*, 312(7023): 71–2.

Straus, S. & Jones, G. 2004, 'What has evidence-based medicine done for us?', *British Medical Journal*, 329(7473): 987–8.

Traynor, M. 2002, 'The oil crisis, risk and evidence-based practice', *Nursing Inquiry*, 9(3): 162–9.

Winch, C., Creedy, D. & Chaboyer, W. 2002, 'Governing nursing conduct: the rise of evidence based practice', *Nursing Inquiry*, 9(3): 156–61.

Index

From the extensive list of books from Ausmed Publications, the publisher especially recommends the following as being of interest to readers of *Wound Care Nursing: A Guide to Practice*.

All of these titles are available from the publisher: Ausmed Publications, 277 Mt Alexander Road, Ascot Vale, Melbourne, Victoria 3032, Australia.

website: <www.ausmed.com.au>; email: <ausmed@ausmed.com.au>

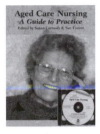

Aged Care Nursing: A Guide to Practice
Edited by Susan Carmody and Sue Forster

The aged population has grown markedly throughout the world, but there is a shortage of experienced nurses with expertise in the holistic care of the elderly. This book is written to inspire and empower such nurses. *Aged Care Nursing: A Guide to Practice* is written by clinicians for clinicians. The inclusion of evidence-based and outcome-based practices throughout the book ensures that all readers, be they novices or experts, will have a reliable and comprehensive reference to guide their practice. Each author is a recognised expert in his or her subject area, and all present their topics with a focus that is practical, rather than academic. Available as textbook alone or as audiobook–textbook package.

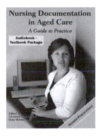

Nursing Documentation in Aged Care: A Guide to Practice
Edited by Christine Crofton and Gaye Witney

The title of this book is carefully chosen. All of the contributors to *Nursing Documentation in Aged Care: A Guide to Practice* firmly believe that nursing documentation in aged care—if performed with pride and professionalism—is truly a *guide to practice*. Documentation is a wonderful opportunity to record and reflect upon all that is good in nursing. In addition to their ethical and professional responsibilities, caring nurses are aware of the personal satisfaction to be gained from documenting their holistic and reflective nursing practice. This book shows how nursing assessments, care plans, and progress notes can allow nurses to share their knowledge, observations, and skills. This is more than a 'how-to-do-it' workbook. With contributions from a range of experts, this comprehensive evidence-based textbook explores the issues surrounding documentation and reveals the importance of professional communication within multidisciplinary teams. Available as textbook alone or as audiobook–textbook package.

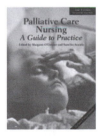

Palliative Care Nursing: A Guide to Practice (2nd edn)
Edited by Margaret O'Connor and Sanchia Aranda

This second edition of Palliative Care Nursing has been totally revised, rewritten, and redesigned. The result is a comprehensive handsome volume that builds upon the successful formula of the popular first edition. All nurses and other health professionals with an interest in this vital subject will welcome this new edition as an essential addition to their libraries. This is the definitive textbook on palliative-care nursing.

From the extensive list of books from Ausmed Publications, the publisher especially recommends the following as being of interest to readers of *Wound Care Nursing: A Guide to Practice*.
All of these titles are available from the publisher: Ausmed Publications, 277 Mt Alexander Road, Ascot Vale, Melbourne, Victoria 3032, Australia.
website: <www.ausmed.com.au>; email: <ausmed@ausmed.com.au>

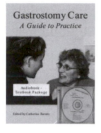

Gastrostomy Care: A Guide to Practice
Edited by Catherine Barrett

The development of the relatively safe PEG procedure has led to a staggering increase in the number of people who receive tube feeding. As another volume in Ausmed's acclaimed 'Guide to Practice' series, *Gastrostomy Care: A Guide to Practice* provides expert practical support for health professionals and family members who care for people who require tube feeding. An important theme of the book is that tube feeding is more than formulae and equipment. People can be devastated to learn that they will no longer be able to eat and drink normally. In adjusting to the personal and social challenges involved, patients and their families require compassion and understanding. This book will assist carers and families to understand the needs of a person with a gastrostomy tube. It provides guidance in managing those needs appropriately, and will assist patients to make informed choices about their tube feeding. Available as textbook alone or as audiobook–textbook package.

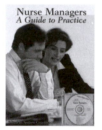

Nurse Managers: A Guide to Practice
Edited by Andrew Crowther

This book addresses the core issues associated with nurse management, and is thus an essential primary text for all nurses as they develop their managerial skills. This book is an innovative and practical text that fulfils a previously unmet need. It provides the evidence-based, practical advice that nurse managers require to undertake their important role with growing confidence and expertise. The book covers such issues as promotion, leadership and motivation, moral management, dealing with unhelpful staff, occupational health and safety, budgets, information technology, and many other vital issues in modern nurse management. In all these areas, the reader is offered a range of solutions and coping strategies for the issues that confront nurse managers every day. Available as textbook alone or as audiobook–textbook package.

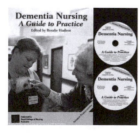

Dementia Nursing: A Guide to Practice
Edited by Rosalie Hudson

Dementia is one of the major health problems of our ageing society and dementia nursing is one of the most important and highly skilled of nursing specialities. As another volume in Ausmed's growing 'Guide to Practice' series, this is the definitive textbook on dementia nursing. The chapters are written primarily by nurses for nurses. But dementia nursing is essentially an exercise in teamwork, and valuable contributions and insights are offered by other health professionals, carers, artists, and relatives from a variety of backgrounds and countries. The result is a comprehensive international volume on all aspects of dementia nursing. Available as textbook alone or as audiobook–textbook package.